Stroke Recovery

An Ultimate Solution to Quick Stroke Recovery

(The Ultimate Guide to a Holistic Approach to Brain Attack Wellness)

Enrique Nelson

Published By **Elena Holly**

Enrique Nelson

Stroke Recovery: An Ultimate Solution to Quick Stroke Recovery (The Ultimate Guide to a Holistic Approach to Brain Attack Wellness)

ISBN   978-1-7770427-1-4

No part of this guidebook shall be reproduced in any form without permission in writing from the publisher except in the case of brief quotations embodied in critical articles or reviews.

Legal & Disclaimer

Table Of Contents

Chapter 1: Movements Of The Hip

AND KNEE JOINTS

The Hip

The hip is a ball and socket joint. These joints allow multidirectional movement and

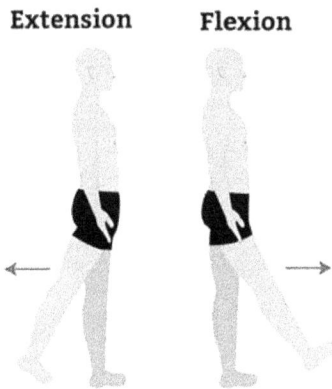

Extension   Flexion

rotation.

Hip flexion and Extension

The hip/joint moreover actions in circumduction. This is moving the leg in a round motion. To carry out this spherical movement, it calls for flexion, extension, abduction, and adduction of the hip.

Notice the foot positioning because the hip performs each movement. Stabilizing the center, pelvic, and hips is crucial to healing the leg, knee, and foot challenges after a stroke.

The knee joint is a hinge joint, and it permits the leg to increase and bend at the knee.

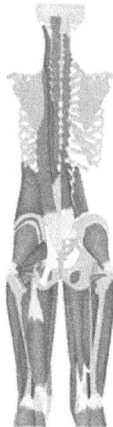

The example of the muscle tissues above indicates some of the severa muscle tissue involved in taking walks and status.

The hips, pelvic, and the trunk of the frame need to end up strong preserving the body upright inside the proper posture for the legs and arms to move freely thru the severa levels of motions and moves they had been made to perform.

As you check the unique hip moves inside the illustrations within the previous pages, you could see that if the hips aren't solid, those movements may be tougher to perform at their complete sort of motion preferred for on foot and particular normal sports.

In the gluteus example, you may see the massive glute muscle and the smaller muscle groups which might be under. The big glute muscle extends the femur, that's the backswing of the leg at the same time as strolling. It moreover rotates the femur outward. The smaller institution of muscle corporations paintings collectively to rotate the femur outward. The femur is the huge better leg bone.

We have a gluteus maximus, medius, and minimus. The gluteus maximus extends the femur and rotates it outward even as the gluteus medius and minimus abducts and rotates the femur inward.

The glute muscle companies are immensely effective. In strolling, they whole the backward motion of the step. When someone has "dishevelled butt," because of this, prone, non-toned, or non-bolstered glutes, this indicates that the glute muscle organizations are not performing their primary characteristic in on foot.

If the spine and lower back muscle groups are prone and there is horrific posture, the hips and pelvic will no longer be robust and stable enough to allow the ones muscle mass and unique muscle tissues much like the piriformis and the opportunity hip rotator muscle agencies which you see in this situation to artwork well. This leaves the spine and again muscular tissues to try and help in those muscle agencies' jobs, leaving the body seeking to feature and flow out of balance, causing ache, weak spot, and harm within the lower back as well as hips, knees, and ankles. Therefore, posture is crucial.

As you keep through this e-book, you may see one of a kind muscle mass concerned in on foot. Studies show that over 70 percentage of the frame's muscle mass are worried in walking.

Gluteus Maximus: Attaches on the ilium and sacrum and to the femur. It extends and rotates the femur outward.

Gluteus Medius: Attaches on the ilium in a twist to the femur. It abducts and rotates the femur inward.

Gluteus Minimus: Attaches on the ilium in a twist to the femur. It abducts and rotates the femur inward.

Piriformis: Attaches on the ischium and the sacrum and to the femur. It rotates the femur outward.

Reminders and suggestions.

When the hip is became round out, this is at the same time because the foot appears. Correcting the foot turn out, foot drag, and foot drop begin inside the hips.

There are 4 quadriceps muscle mass. They are the vastus intermedius, rectus femoris, vastus medialis, and the vastus lateralis.

They are muscular tissues of the the front of the thigh. The quadriceps assists increase and pushes ahead the thigh and leg while taking walks.

The Sartorius is the longest muscle within the body. It is connected to the front of the ilium, crosses over the medial difficulty of the thigh, and from the knee to the the the the front of the tibia. Although it is an anterior muscle, it inserts into the tibia from within the lower back of the knee, and it flexes the foreleg. It additionally flexes, abducts, and laterally rotates the thigh on the hip. The greater survivors, caregivers, and experts comprehend about the muscle tissues of the frame and the movements they carry out, the higher risk they've got in strengthening the frame accurately to help in in addition and more potent recovery. The sartorius lets in to raise the leg in taking steps at the equal time as strolling.

Sartorius: Attaches at the ilium and crosses over the medial difficulty of the thigh inside the back of the knee, then join at the tibia. It flexes the foreleg. It is also inside the institution of hip flexor muscle corporations. This is the longest muscle on the frame.

Popliteus: Attaches on the femur and the tibia. It flexes the foreleg and rotates it inward. It allows at unlocking the knee so it can flex. The popliteus is established in a later example in this e-book.

Tensor Fasciae Latae: Attaches to the ilium, patella, and tibia. It flexes and abducts the femur.

Tibia: is one of the decrease leg bones. The specific is the Fibula. The Tibia is the larger of those bones

Fibula: is one of the lower leg bones. The distinct is the Tibia. The Fibula is the thinner of these bones.

Ilium: is the most important a part of the hip bone and the better part of the hip bone.

Ischium: is the posterior/inferior location of the hip bone. It permits the body at the same time as sitting.

Quadriceps: way 4 heads.

Patella is the kneecap bone.

Pectineus attaches to the pubis and to the femur. It flexes the femur.

Gracilis Attaches to the pubic bone and goes within the returned of the knee and then attaches to the the front of the tibia. It adducts the hip, flexes the knee, and flexes the foreleg.

Adductor Magnus attaches to the pubis, ischium, and the once more of the femur.

Adductor Brevis attaches to the pubis and femur. It adducts the femur.

Adductor Longus attaches to the pubis and the femur. It adducts the femur.

Adductor Minimus (NOT mounted in example) It attaches to the pubis and the femur and adducts the femur.

All adductor muscle groups inside the thighs pull the legs closer to the middle of the body when walking. This allows hold balance.

Chapter 2: Hyper Extended Knee
AND FOOT DROP

A hyperextended knee is at the same time as the knee is driven beyond its ordinary form of movement bypassing the right away role. This can be not unusual for loads stroke survivors. The sports on this e-book and my motion pictures can assist recuperation a hyperextended knee. BUT the CORE MUST BE STRONG TO STABILIZE THE PELVIC GIRDLE AND HIPS. I positioned that closing sentence in bold because of the fact if the center is prone, the hips and pelvic girdle may be susceptible and unstable whilst sitting and standing. There are tons an awful lot much less threat that the knee will heal inside the ones activities.

If the hips are not placed well, the knee cannot be well positioned to perform the proper actions. I stated in advance within the ebook

Popliteus: Attaches at the femur and the tibia. It flexes the foreleg and rotates it inward. It helps at unlocking the knee in order that it could flex. The popliteus is verified in a later example on this book.

Foot drop is also referred to as drop foot. I moreover am searching for advice from it as foot drop and leg drag. This is even as it is hard to reinforce the the the the front a part of the foot. The bodily video games on this e-book and my movies can assist restore foot drop. BUT THE CORE MUST BE STRONG TO STABILIZE THE PELVIC GIRDLE AND HIPS. I located that remaining sentence in ambitious due to the fact if the center is inclined, the hips and pelvic girdle can also be prone and risky whilst sitting and status, and the foot drop cannot successfully heal.

Movements that raise the foot off the ground start inside the hips and higher legs, now not the foot.

THE FOOT AND ANKLE

It is common for stroke survivors to have annoying situations with strolling. One of the annoying situations is making an attempt to get better topics in conjunction with drop foot, spasticity, numbness, and additional.

Remember that in case you are clearly appearing sporting occasions to work the lower leg muscle groups to move the foot within the ones specific movements, it's going to not create the whole movements had to carry the leg, bend the knee and take a step for on foot. The middle and trunk of the frame need to be robust and sturdy to hold the hips and pelvic in right alignment. This is important to assist the body so that the muscle mass that flex and enlarge the hip, thigh, knee, and foot can carry out the motion that takes a step to stroll.

Soleus: Attaches to the back of the tibia and the again of the calcaneus. It extends the ankle and foot.

Gastrocnemius: Attaches to the again of the femur and the again of the calcaneus. It extends the ankle and foot.

Calcaneus: The heel bone.

Malleolus: A bony detail at the factor of the ankle

Plantaris: Attaches to the once more of the femur and the yet again of the calcaneus. It extends the ankle and foot. This muscle isn't always classified in the illustrations on this e-book.

Flexor Hallucis Longus: Attaches to the back of the fibula and is going within the again of the ankle and below the foot to the cease of the huge toe. This toe is referred to as the toe primary. It extends the ankle and foot. This muscle is not labeled inside the illustrations in this book.

Flexor Digitorum Longus: Attaches to the lower back of the tibia and goes within the lower back of the ankle and beneath the foot to the give up of four of the five toes. It does now not attach to the massive toe. It extends the ankle and foots this muscle in not labeled in the illustrations in this e-book.

Tibialis Posterior: Attaches to the lower returned of the tibia and is going at the back of the malleolus and beneath the foot to the 3 middle metatarsals. It extends and adducts the foot. This muscle isn't always classified in the illustrations on this e-book.

Peroneus Longus: Attaches to the fibula and is going inside the again of the malleolus and beneath the foot to the bottom of the big toe. It extends and abducts the foot. This muscle isn't classified within the illustrations in this e-book.

Peroneus Brevis: Attaches to the fibula and is going inside the again of the malleolus to the lowest of the pinky toe. It extends and abducts the foot. This muscle isn't always categorised within the illustrations in this e-book.

Extension of the ankle and foot is at the same time as we stand on our tiptoes. It is also the place whilst we are sitting down and pointing the ft away from the frame.

Flexion of the ankle and foot is whilst we're reputation flat on our ft. It is also positing when we're sitting down, pulling the feet in the course of the body.

Did you apprehend that having tight calves can add to shoulder, hip, and lower again pain, further to movement problems? Remember that the fascia intertwines thru the entire body.

At the the the the the front of the decrease leg, there are the tibialis muscles. These enhance the foot as one takes a taking walks stride the maintain the foot up in order that it does not scrape the floor in steps. Walking and education taking walks permits keep those muscle groups strengthened for on foot. Not all leg muscle tissues are mounted on this example.

Tibialis Anterior: Attaches to the the the the front of the tibia and the lowest of the extended bone in the once more of the massive toe. This will be the metatarsal number one; it flexes and adducts the ankle and foot. This muscle is not categorised within the illustrations on this e-book.

Extensor Hallucis Longus: Attaches to the front of the fibula and the stop of the large toe. It Flexes the Ankle and foot. This muscle isn't classified inside the illustrations in this book.

Extensor digitorum Longus: Attaches to the the the front of the fibula and the ends of the variety to 5 ft. It does not attach to the huge toe. It flexes the ankle and foot. This muscle is not categorized inside the illustrations on this ebook.

Chapter 3: Strengthening The Postural

MUSCLES IS ESSENTIAL FOR

STANDING AND WALKING

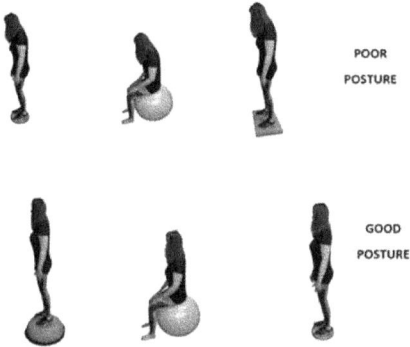

POOR POSTURE

GOOD POSTURE

Posture is essential. These images of posture may additionally moreover furthermore appearance acquainted to you when you have check my special books. I need to percent visuals to help you become privy to your posture while you sit down, stand, and stroll.

This economic spoil has pretty some statistics, and it can be overwhelming for a few. As a stroke survivor, you do now not have to memorize all the understanding and muscle groups. This monetary smash is right proper right here to teach and offer visuals and a extra statistics of muscle groups and movements to assist assist you better to a stronger healing. I experience facts is energy.

Studies show communique a number of the spinal twine to each the mind and the limbs can be compromised if the backbone or spinal cord is in bad posture. See the pix of my horrible posture. The hip and pelvic girdle cannot be sturdy and stable to help the leg muscle groups, which want to gain the power required to benefit a more potent restoration in the legs and strolling gait. This consists of supporting restore foot drop and leg drag. In a few survivors, the affected leg feels very heavy, and a few have numb spots and no feeling in areas.

When someone stands rounded over with the hips tucked underneath, as seen within the pics of me, it limits the form of movement the legs must make in movements collectively with taking walks. Poor posture also indicates that there are susceptible center, spine, and once more muscle agencies. When this takes location, exceptional muscle organizations try and do the manner of these postural muscle corporations, main to greater malfunction.

An important tip on the identical time as performing your bodily therapy and/or schooling (exercising) on posture, balance, popularity, and walking talents is to hold your eyes searching in advance. Your body follows your eyeballs. If you appearance or face down, the body will try and observe. It will maintain you in horrible posture.

The pelvis's stabilizing muscle tissue have to be robust and in balance. These muscles are also essential in strolling. You will have a look at some of those muscle tissues inside the path of this e-book.

The first photo indicates my client leaning slightly ahead. This will not purpose the body to rebuild new pathways, the strength, nor the cognitive abilities needed to rebuild stability and spatial reputation this is required to be stable in repute, taking walks, and regular actions. Also, all the muscle groups are not building strength inside the positions needed to help unique muscle companies additionally assemble the power they need. Studies display that after the body is in right posture, all the abilties and systems artwork better. In the second one picture, she is upright. In this role, the deep spinal muscle tissues can be activated properly to help build the strength and proprioception wished for more solid mobility and stabilization in motion.

She is operating on her postural muscle mass and her balance in proper alignment within the 2d photograph. Note: She has a bar on the wall for safety. I propose normally having a bar and a consistent environment on your workout and balancing practices. Safety First!

Also, if you look closely at those snap shots, you could see that she is repute at the BOSU® ball in a single picture and a stability pad inside the unique. As from my teachings and books, those are every brilliant balance machine even as used very well and nicely.

In the subsequent four illustrations, I show some of the muscular tissues on the way to not paintings to their great commonplace normal performance needed for walking if the frame is leaning earlier, as visible within the illustration of the man leaning ahead to walk.

The example above is on an excessive thoughts-set. This is for coaching capabilities to assist deliver a imaginative and prescient of at the same time as the frame does no longer line up in right posture from head to toe, it reasons more worrying conditions.

Here is a brief section on some of the center muscle corporations. I moreover like to consult them due to the fact the postural muscle groups and the stabilizing device.

The spine ismade up of

7 cervical vertebrae,

12 thoracic vertebrae,

5 lumbar vertebrae.

The sacrum is five vertebrae fused together.

At the bottom of the sacrum is the coccyx, that is known as the tail bone (Not seen in this instance).

The manner I undergo in mind the type of vertebrae is with the resource of something that my university professor taught me.

"We devour breakfast at 7:00, lunch at 12:00 and dinner at five: 00."

If you have got were given study my books, some of what I will percentage approximately the psoas muscle may additionally sound familiar. The psoas is a vital muscle placed in the center of the body. It lies deep beneath the transverse belly muscle. It is a deep lower back muscle, and it is the great spinal muscle that proper now attaches to the legs. The psoas muscle is the handiest muscle inside the decrease again that crosses over the hips and attaches on the the the the front of the body. It attaches to the remaining thoracic vertebrae and 4 of the five lumbar vertebrae and on the femur, the top thigh bone. It is likewise the bridge a number of the hips and the again. The psoas is frequently referred to as the iliopsoas. This is even as the psoas and the iliacus muscle organizations are being grouped in discussions.

The psoas and the iliacus are of the three muscle tissues that help solid the low backbone to the pelvis. The quadratus lumborum is the 1/three muscle.

If the belly muscle businesses (a part of the center muscles) are vulnerable, the psoas tries to perform the paintings of the stomach muscle agencies. If the psoas is brief, susceptible, and/or tight, it will possibly be tough to hold the body in an upright position with the shoulders stacked over the hips. Also, there can be more of a assignment for a stroke survivor if the psoas has spasticity in any of its fibers. Spasticity does no longer best take vicinity within the arm and legs. It can upward push up in any muscle in the frame.

For instance, if there can be spasticity in a unmarried or some of the multifidus or spinal rotatores, it can make it more difficult to work on posture, balance, and stabilization of the spine and body. This is every other reason to hold working on strengthening the middle and postural muscle tissues. See my different books, Stroke Recovery, What Now? When Physical Therapy Ends, But Your Recovery Continues. It has a financial ruin on center and spine muscle tissue plus a chapter on sports, and the ebook The Power of Your Spine, How Back Strength and Posture Pilots the Entire Body.

Multifidus

The multifidus is a small but effective muscle. It is the number one stabilizing muscle of the backbone. This muscle takes the strain off the vertebral discs simply so the body weight can be allotted in the course of the spine. If this is inclined, you will moreover have weak spot in the low decrease decrease lower back. The multifidus begins offevolved to activate in advance than the frame moves to guard the spine. It is a part of the stabilizing device in the body. The multifidus is also one of the muscle groups within the backbone that extends, abducts, adducts, and rotates the spine. To gain a better stability, this muscle needs to be sturdy. Performing diverse physical activities combining with the Swiss ball, stability disc, and BOSU® ball will help benefit a stronger multifidus. Better posture ends in a better stability. See my books, Tipping toward Balance or Stroke Recovery What Now? For bodily sports on balance and stabilization.

To help this sound less difficult, at the same time as we bend over from the spine (rounding the backbone), the movement is known as spinal flexion. When we are moving the spine from flexed function lower again as much as being upright, it is called spinal extension, additionally referred to as Axial Extension. Flexion is at the same time as a muscle brings joints together. An extension is taking the 2 joints farther aside. For example, even as we flex our arm to reveal our arm muscle mass (the bicep) as in acting a bicep curl exercising, that is flexion. As you enlarge the arm decrease again out right away, it's far an extension.

The small muscle tissues close to the vertebrae need to be activated harmoniously. These muscle businesses are postural muscle groups. Exercising on a volatile floor, in conjunction with the Swiss ball, balance disc, and the BOSU® ball stimulates the relevant nervous gadget, which might be the thoughts and the spinal cord. It strengthens muscular tissues and ligaments, in addition to activating and strengthening all of the small muscles alongside the spinal column.

The multifidus muscle, transverse belly muscle, diaphragm, and the pelvic ground muscle businesses are all on the identical neuromuscular loop. This manner it is first rate if those forms of muscle groups are functioning well; each desires to carry out its interest for my part and as a collection. Stated a bit extra complex, it manner a sequential segmental neuromuscular stimulation with closed-loop remarks. If the transverse muscle is inclined, the pelvic ground, the multifidus, and the diaphragm can't benefit right strength to perform their jobs in a healthy, functioning frame.

Often stroke survivors want to enhance and correct their posture. Even for seniors and others with balance and stabilization issues, gaining robust postural muscle mass is critical. Proper posture need to be strengthened to assist the alternative stabilizing muscle tissue to maintain the body strongly upright so it may reap a posture wherein the shoulders are stacked over the hips. If the pinnacle is upright and balanced over the shoulders, we've a better stability. The balance inside the pelvis and hips must be made just so the decrease limbs and joints can benefit power, function in alignment, and perform properly for safe moves.

Transverse Abdominal Muscle

The transverse muscle is the internal maximum of the stomach muscle mass. This isn't always a backbone or once more muscle, however if this muscle isn't strong, the multifidus backbone muscle cannot be robust. The transverse muscle's crucial characteristic is to stabilize the lower once more and pelvis earlier than motion. It is the non-public belly muscle, wrapping across the frame to behave like a corset. It allows stabilize the hips and pelvic. When engaged, it furthermore pulls the stomach in and offers help to the thoracolumbar fascia. It is the stabilizer of the shoulder girdle, the pinnacle, neck, pelvis, and decrease extremities.

For those who are looking for to accurate posture or are in rehabilitation to discover ways to stand and stroll again or a person who has rounded shoulders and negative posture, it's miles vital to reinforce this muscle. It need to be reinforced to help the possibility stabilizing muscle agencies to keep the frame strongly upright so that it could benefit a posture in which the shoulders are stacked over the hips. If the top is upright and balanced over the shoulders, we've got were given have been given a higher balance. The stability in the pelvis and hips need to be made simply so the decrease limbs and joints can benefit electricity, characteristic in alignment, and carry out well for secure moves.

Before we flow into ahead to every other muscle, I desire it is becoming clearer to you genuinely how muscle groups art work collectively to assist one-of-a-kind muscle corporations inside the frame carry out their jobs.

The pelvic floor muscular tissues artwork as stabilizers of the stomach and pelvic organs The pelvic floor muscles and the gluteus (buttock) muscle businesses are made to art work and go together with the waft in opposite guidelines. One must be able to have interaction the pelvic floor without engaging the gluteus muscle groups to advantage pinnacle-rated center electricity. These muscle tissues should be separated inside the brain and aggravating system for everyday body functioning. This moreover plays a function in preventing back troubles. The transverse muscle should be robust for the pelvic ground to come to be robust and feature properly thinking about the reality that they're on the equal neuromuscular loop.

Reminders and tips.

In every one in each of my books, I percentage this inside the anatomy segment:

The transverse stomach muscle, the multifidus muscle, diaphragm, and the pelvic floor muscular tissues are all at the identical neuromuscular loop. This manner it's far extraordinary if these types of muscle tissues are functioning well; each wants to perform its mission personally and as a collection. If the transverse muscle is inclined, the pelvic floor, the multifidus, and the diaphragm cannot benefit right electricity to carry out their jobs for a healthy, functioning body.

The Other Abdominal Muscles

The transverse abdominals had been cited in advance inside the ebook. Now permit us to test the opposite 3 belly muscle tissue.

Rectus Abdominus

The rectus abdominus is the maximum superficial belly muscle. This is the muscle that creates the "six-percentage" appearance. It attaches on the the front of the ribs 5 through 7 and to the pubis. It flexes and adducts the spine. It permits the tilt of the pelvis and the curvature of the low spine. It moreover adducts the ribs causing exhalation. Often while human beings simply do belly crunches and no actual beneficial training of the abs and center, this muscle can get tight, adding or inflicting lower back ache.

Internal Oblique

The word oblique, steady with the Oxford Dictionary, manner neither parallel nor a proper mindset to a line, however slanting at an perspective. Both the internal and out of doors indirect muscle fibers run on an attitude.

The inner indirect is on the lateral (difficulty) thing of the trunk. It attaches at ribs 10 thru 12 and to the crest of the ilium (pelvic bone). It adducts the ribs, inflicting exhalation. It additionally flexes, abducts, and adducts and rotates the backbone.

External Oblique

The external indirect attaches from rib 5 through 12 and to the crest of the ilium It adducts the ribs, inflicting exhalation and flexes, adducts, and rotates the spine.

If the deep backbone muscle businesses which you look at approximately in advance on this ebook are willing and now not performing their activity nicely, those outer muscle groups will pull tougher at the spine, which could result in damage and malfunction. It is particularly crucial to decorate the body from the interior out, similar to a little one develops. This is a key to balance, spine and again care, proprioception, stabilization, and protection of the spine. It is likewise the important detail to constructing all the spine and center muscle companies to their top notch energy so all of the muscle tissues can consciousness on handiest the activity they had been made to do. This moreover leaves the body a tremendous deal a lot much less fatigued.

Abdominal muscles settlement with each step at the same time as we stroll.

In the example above, the proper aspect indicates sections tremendous for learning capabilities. They aren't interested in their complete attachments sooner or later of the whole spine.

The Transversospinalis organization consists of:

The rotators, interspinales, and intertransversarii.

These muscle agencies are critical for providing proprioception feedback most of the thoughts, lower back, and entire frame.

Rotators - The hobby of those muscles is to boom the backbone and rotation to the other detail. It movements with proprioception, bringing balance at the same time as the frame is in movement. They are the personal and most medial layer of spinal fascial. They boom the spine and rotation to the opportunity aspect. This business enterprise of muscle groups has loads to do with proprioception, mainly the rotators and the interspinales. The interspinales has lots to do with the comments some of the again and mind and from the mind to the lower lower back. They are the internal maximum (deeper than the multifidus) and have the maximum medial layer of spinal fascia. "Medial" technique it's far the closest to the middle of the frame.

Interspinales – Move the spine in segmental extension. This muscle brings pretty a few proprioception for the decrease back, stability, and stability of the spine and body in motion.

Intertransversarii – Moves the spine in small segmental motions and lateral flexion of the spine.

They are small muscles which are probably on each sides of the backbone.

The Interspinales and Intertransversarii muscle mass pass and stabilize the spine. They additionally play an essential position in body cognizance and proprioception.

Therefore, it is so essential to boost the center and backbone from the inner out. The frame communicates from movement and movements, starting deep inside the spine. This is why after I educate clients to regain their functionality and cognitive abilities, which encompass stability, spatial hobby, and proprioception, I begin with easy however particularly effective bodily video video games like reputation on stability discs, stability pads, and/or BOSU® balls. This enables rebuild those muscular tissues and their herbal verbal exchange to the thoughts and once more.

Quadratus Lumborum

The quadratus lumborum (QL) (as you can see within the illustrations) attaches from the lumbar vertebrae and rib 12 to the crest of the ilium. It stabilizes the pelvis (hip girdle) at the same time as walking and laterally flexes the backbone. It has three layers of fibers that flow into in 3 precise suggestions. The quadratus lumborum can reason masses of pain. When this muscle is best activated (or in spasticity) on one factor, the trunk is bent in the direction of that path. The QL is one of the muscle groups that help solid the low backbone to the pelvis.

As you may see interior the instance of the quadratus lumborum, the only the right shows that if one issue of the QT is shorter than the other facet, it is able to hike up the pelvis/hips. This could have an effect on the whole body. It may additionally have an effect on shoulder joint and arm moves moreover.

When a person sits with their hips off to at least one factor, this imbalance will take region to extraordinary deep muscle tissue of the backbone as nicely. This includes the psoas muscle.

For example, if a person is trying to observe to stroll once more, and they spend lots time sitting with the muscular tissues on this function. When they stand or stroll, they'll not have the electricity, balance, and muscle connection to regain the talent at their brilliant. These illustrations are also another seen to expose the electricity of the backbone muscle businesses.

The customers who artwork on their posture anywhere they go, now not truly whilst they are with me, get the tremendous consequences.

Chapter 4: The Spinal Engine

WORKING THROUGH THE FASCIA

LINES THEORIES

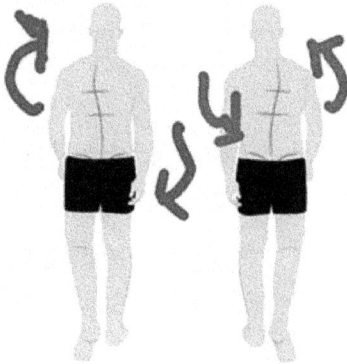

The Spinal Engine Theory

Above, you could see that when the left arm swings forward, the higher backbone rotates ahead at the left due to the fact the right hip rotates over again because the backbone rotates for taking walks steps. This follows the Spinal Engine Theory, which I believe is the first-class idea. The spine rotates as we walk.

The thoracolumbar fascia enables the decrease lower back muscle groups and permits them achieve the functionality to transport the body. It is made from robust fibers and permits channel forces of movement because the once more muscle tissues settlement and loosen up. The nerves to the ones muscular tissues also skip through this fascia. This fascia is going deep to the spine and is fabricated from 3 layers. It is important for contralateral motions like taking walks. It works with the latissimus dorsi (lats) to coil the middle of the body.

When the thoracolumbar fascia is supported, it lets in all of the muscle businesses that connect with it to function better. These muscle groups encompass the gluteus maximus, latissimus dorsi, trapezius, erector spine, quadratus lumborum, psoas, transverse, and inner obliques. It helps bridge the muscle groups of the decrease lower lower back to the muscular tissues of the stomach wall. This fascia facilitates to integrate the moves of the higher frame with the decrease body. Nerves from seven particular muscle mass in the center run via the thoracolumbar fascia.

Latissimus Dorsi: Attaches at the hip and the low decrease again and to the humerus.

It extends, adducts, and rotates inward the humerus. It attaches into the thoracolumbar fascia. It additionally adducts, extends, and medially rotates the humerus.

See more about the electricity of the backbone muscle tissues and the thoracolumbar fascia in my books The Power of Your Spine, How Back Strength and Posture Pilots the Entire Body and Stroke Recovery What Now? When Physical Therapy Ends, But Your Recovery Continues.

In this example, you could see the large glute muscle businesses and the smaller muscle tissues which is probably under. As proven previously on this ebook with categorized muscle businesses, the big glute muscle extends the femur, this is the backswing of the leg at the identical time as on foot. It additionally rotates the femur outward. The smaller institution of muscular tissues art work together to rotate the femur outward.

The left latissimus dorsi art work with the right glutes and vice versa in actions, and taking walks.

The core want to get more potent for the backbone to get its herbal rotation decrease once more for a wholesome taking walks gait. Walking starts offevolved offevolved offevolved on the middle.

The Myofascial Lines

I will percent a totally quick description of the myofascial lines. I furthermore percentage some illustrations to provide an photo that will help you higher recognize movement and how every vicinity of the body could have an effect on the alternative

The myofascial lines act to exchange the pulling pressure of one muscle to the opportunity muscle businesses in the body which might be connected with every fascial line(s) worried. These myofascial strains are also defined as a line that transmits pulling forces sooner or later of the frame. As Thomas Myers teaches in his e-book, Anatomy Trains, this pulling pressure, moreover called anxiety, transfers sequentially from one myofascial unit of the traces to the subsequent. It has been described to be just like the dominoes impact. I substantially advocate if you are within the fitness corporation, a bodily therapist, a rub down therapist, or different recuperation experts, to have a look at the e-book Anatomy Trains and teachings by using manner of Thomas Myers.

In stroke restoration, I experience that is fantastic records to help survivors and caregivers to understand extra about how, for instance, a few element taking place within the shoulder may also have an impact on or limit the moves or restoration of the hip and foot, and so forth. There are many connections through the frame like this.

There are many greater illustrations to train the ones fascial lines. I am simply sharing some of them in this e-book. This can be complex, so I am leaving it clean on this e book and advocate reading extra approximately it in your personal and looking at the severa different illustrations to be had.

FASCIA

Fascia is a non-stop form that surrounds and intermingles tissues and structures for the duration of the frame. It varies in density and thickness. Nerves and blood vessels moreover run through the fascia. When the thoughts is sending messages for movement, it consists of the fascia. Training survivors with statistics of fascia is essential on the identical time as deciding on which bodily sports are the brilliant for each person. Fascia is likewise interconnected with the structures it surrounds. The health and mobility of fascia play a massive characteristic in the body to have healthful movement and to avoid ache and harm. There are ongoing studies on fascia and its obligatory importance for the frame to transport.

"Fascia consists of mechanoreceptors and proprioceptors. In different terms, each time we use a muscle, we stretch fascia that is related to spindle cells, Ruffini and Paccini corpuscles, and Golgi organs. The regular stretching of fascia consequently communicates the strain of the muscle contraction and the repute of the muscle concerning its tone, movement, charge of change in muscle duration, and feature of the associated frame element to the valuable involved system." From Dr. Warren Hammer, the chiropractic profession's leading expert in soft tissues and fascia, "The Fascial System is a Sensory Organ."

Dr. Hammer went on to say in any other article, "Why We Need to Fix the Mechanoreceptors" that, "One of the maximum applicable discoveries within the worldwide of anatomy over those many years is that muscle spindles, the chief proprioceptive cells affecting our muscle tissues, are not inside the muscle, however in the fascia surrounding the muscle and its muscle bundles A mechanoreceptor is stimulated at the same time as its miles deformed, but whilst it's far restrained in the fascia this is not capable of go with the waft. It is not able to stretch, this is important for the function of the spindle cell."

The thoracolumbar fascia is an crucial fascia to recognize. It is crucial for walking, walking, and mobility. The thoracolumbar fascia helps the decrease again muscles and lets in them collect the capability to transport the frame. It is made of strong fibers and permits channel forces of motion because of the reality the back muscle groups agreement and loosen up, that is important for contralateral motions like on foot. The nerves to those muscle groups additionally circulate through this fascia. This fascia goes deep to the spine and is fabricated from three layers. It works with the latissimus dorsi (lats) to coil the center of the frame.

When the thoracolumbar fascia is supported, it lets in all of the muscular tissues that connect with it function better. These muscle groups encompass the gluteus maximus, latissimus dorsi, trapezius, erector backbone, quadratus lumborum, psoas, transverse stomach, and inner obliques. It enables bridge the muscle tissue of the decrease lower back to the muscular tissues of the belly wall. This fascia allows integrate the movements of the pinnacle body with the decrease frame.

Chapter 5: The Sciatic Nerve

As running shoes and therapists, even as we pay hobby "sciatic nerve," we right away assume ache. Although the sciatic nerve is stated to be the biggest unmarried nerve within the body, it is fabricated from five nerves. It is positioned at the proper and left facet of the decrease backbone thru the fourth and fifth lumbar nerves and the primary three nerves in the sacral spine. At the largest a part of the nerve, it is as big as a male thumb. The 5 nerves business enterprise at the the the front of the piriformis muscles and come to be one massive nerve, called the sciatic nerve. This nerve additives sensation and strength to the leg and the reflexes of the leg. It connects the spinal twine with the outside of the thigh, the hamstring muscle companies, and the muscular tissues of the lower leg and ft. It offers motor and sensory skills to areas of the leg and foot. When the sciatic nerve is impaired, it may bring about muscle weak point and/or numbness and tingling inside the leg, ankle, foot, and toes. The sciatic nerve and its nerve branches allow movement and feeling in the thigh, knee, calf,

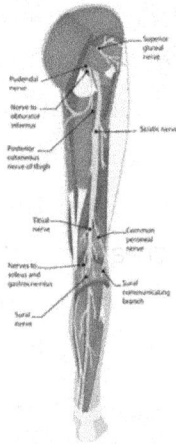

ankle, foot, and ft.

This example indicates the sciatic nerve and its nerve branches.

This sciatic nerve exits the spinal cord some of the 4th and 5th lumbar vertebrae and travels down each elements of the spine and to/through the piriformis muscle companies. Poor posture and slouching as one sits can affect the low backbone and the sciatic nerve. Posture is crucial, even at the equal time as sitting.

Deltoids

The Shoulder

The Anterior head of the Deltoid attaches to the clavicle and the humerus.

The clavicle is the collar bone. It flexes, abducts, and rotates the humerus inward.

The medial head of the Deltoid attaches to the scapula and the humerus. It abducts the humerus.

The posterior head of the Deltoid attaches to the backbone of the scapula and the humerus. It extends, abducts, and rotates the humerus outward.

Sternocleidomastoid attaches to the mastoid device, sternum (breastbone), and clavicle (collar bone). It flexes, abducts, and adducts the backbone.

Reminders and recommendations.

Scapula is the Shoulder blade.

Humerus is the top arm bone.

Clavicle is the collar bone.

Anterior is in the path of the the front.

Medial is inside the middle.

Posterior is towards the decrease decrease again.

Four muscle corporations make up what's known as the "rotator cuff."

These 4 muscle agencies paintings together as a team to hold the shoulder girdle nicely in location just so the shoulder joint can bypass freely and nicely. These 4 muscle agencies are the Supraspinatus, Infraspinatus, Teres Minor, and Subscapularis. They paintings as a crew, but moreover they've movements that they perform one after the other. Using the shoulder joint in sports activities sports and regular sports activities activities in bad posture, will encourage disorder and create an harm. It is not unusual for me to pay attention clients say they have a "rotator cuff harm" and not realize which muscle or ligament it is. Many humans simply anticipate it is a cuff and do now not recognize that 4 muscle groups are growing the so-referred to as "cuff."

Supraspinatus attaches to the scapula and the humerus. It abducts the humerus.

Infraspinatus attaches to the scapula and the humerus. It extends and rotates the humerus outward.

Teres Minor attaches at the scapula and the humerus. It extends and rotates the humerus outward.

Subscapularis attaches to the scapula and the humerus. It adducts and rotates the humerus inward.

As you can see, all 4 muscular tissues hook up with the scapula and the humerus. However, each of those rotator cuff muscle agencies attaches to specific regions of the scapula and certainly one of a type regions of the humerus. To hold it simple, I did now not listing the correct problem of attachment.

The arm and shoulder muscle mass also play a position in on foot. When the hands swing, they devise strength in strolling. When the arms are in swinging motion with strolling, they encourage the spine to do the herbal rotation that performs within the walking movement. This is a few other purpose it's far vital to have accurate posture, so the shoulders are within the proper feature for the hands to swing. In recuperation, regularly, one arm isn't always cooperating inside the moves because of the stroke effect. The hands have a stronger chance of gaining a better recuperation while the shoulders are aligned properly for the shoulder's ball and socket joint to transport freely. This is based totally totally on the frame to be in proper posture.

Reminders and hints.

Adduct approach bringing part of the frame lower again to the midline of the frame.

Abduction manner moving part of the frame further from the midline of the frame.

Rotation outward approach rotating a part of the frame far from the midline of the frame.

Rotation inward method rotating part of the frame lower decrease again towards the midline of the frame.

Muscles that join on the scapula and humerus should be activated to regain arm movement again. This way acting sporting sports and movement treatment that circulate the scapula.

To take a look at greater about the recuperation of the arms, see my ebook, Stroke Recovery, Regaining Arm Movement. This e book has illustrations of the muscle, nerves, and movements, further to recommendations and physical video games covered.

Chapter 6: Having A Safety Bar

FOR EXERCISE

First, I want to remind you of the importance of analyzing the e-book earlier than in reality turning to this monetary disaster to do carrying activities. The cause of my books is to assist educate professionals, caregivers, and stroke survivors approximately muscular tissues, motion, physical video video games, and safety. When you've got an know-how of why a particular exercising is being executed and the way to do it well, there's a higher

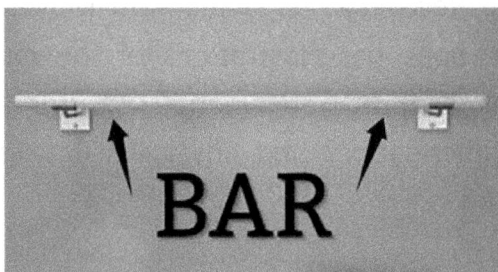

hazard for further restoration.

Second, I need it to be easy that having a bar on a wall to exercising with is an important exercising tool to have in stroke restoration, stability training, and fall prevention.

I count on the length of the bar ought to be at the least 3 ft up to 6 or 8 feet. This will depend upon your place and the capability to have one installed for you. The longer the bar, the farther you could exercise on foot and taking thing steps with it.

One of the motives it's miles best to have a strong bar to apply in comparison to countertops and furnishings to workout with is a bar may be grabbed for protection. A countertop and one-of-a-kind volatile surfaces maintain one at risk to fall, and you are exceptionally confined to what exercise and development you could do. With a bar, you may experience more strong and function a sense of manipulate which you do no longer have without it.

Holing onto the bar and squatting can bring together the talents and energy to stand and help begin to rebuild a robust middle and proper posture. I surely have said severa times in this ebook, and my different books, that a strong center and proper posture is crucial for stability, stabilization, recognition, and on foot. Keeping a chair beneath you for safety and as preferred as you help is vital, as seen inside the following image.

You can put a chair or wheelchair near the bar and exercise status up from seated positions right into a tall, proper posture.

Many survivors can fine use one arm, as seen in the following image. In this situation, it is able to take a survivor longer to benefit the body strength in the popularity and squatting moves due to the truth they satisfactory have one arm to rely upon. Be affected person if you could.

As you upward thrust up from a chair or a squat position, paintings on keeping the hips sturdy with the aid of retaining the ft anchored to the ground, and going via earlier flippantly.

Keep the abs engaged. This will assist hold the hips from swaying to 1 element as those moves are carried out.

Every time you get up, stand up absolutely from head to toe.

Try to maintain toes degree on the floor. Do not let them roll out to the rims. Keep all toes down, if feasible.

You are building the power, balance, talents, and pathways to status up strongly, so on foot can emerge as more potent and greater stable.

On flat surfaces, collectively with counter tops and risky furniture, you have were given had been given nothing to grip onto for protection for you to preserve your body weight.

Another plus to the usage of a bar is as your unaffected hand and affected hand (if and at the equal time as it can) grabs onto the bar, you're the use of your hands for gripping, grabbing, quick reaction time, which builds more potent palms, wrist, arms and finger strength. The hands and toes can start to retrain shifting and coordinating collectively with manage, rebuilding pathways to arms, palms, and hands, and masses greater.

Safety First!

With the hand worrying situations, many survivors face working closer to, gripping, and freeing the affected hand from the bar is proper for arms that grip too much and for the hands a high-quality way to no longer grip the least bit.

As you assessment the only-of-a-type bodily games in this e-book, please take be conscious that now not all survivors are at the same vicinity in restoration. There is probably bodily sports that one survivor can try this some other survivor cannot do. All survivors have to begin at their private vicinity to start and increase at their very personal tempo.

When you be aware the sports activities recognition on stability pads, BOSU® balls and discs, understand to ALWAYS begin popularity at the ground first the use of the bar.

When you are wanting to exercising standing up from a chair or a wheelchair, use the bar. Each time you get up, try and engage your abs and stand without a doubt up.

Many instances, while people are struggling with balance, stabilization, and strolling, they do not entire their upward push up and try to take steps with the body in terrible posture. This makes it greater hard and danger for falls. BUT, if you are having trouble and enjoy UNSAFE, USE THE BAR until you may sense secure and ALWAYS have a person with you to art work with. If possible, find a instructor or therapist to maintain you SAFE.

Standing on a BOSU® ball additionally carrying activities the muscle tissues in Illustration in resistance education. Remember, those muscular tissues assist to hold the femur bone (better thigh bone) upright and solid for reputation and strolling.

Hold on with each fingers, and whilst equipped, you may rotate every hands by manner of using maintaining on with only one hand for some seconds or longer. This will all rely on anyone's non-public case and capability at the time of exercising.

Be positive to maintain onto a strong item which encompass a bar secured to a wall.

Stand in a proper posture with the abs engaged.

If you're doing arm and hand bodily sports activities as shared in my book Stroke Recovery, Gaining Arm Movement, if feasible, do the physical sports activities on the non-affected hand first.

The physical sports shared on this ebook may be performed sitting, standing at the ground, status on BOSU® ball, balance disc, stability pad, kneeling on a BOSU® ball, sitting on a ball, or sitting in a chair. Ensure your protection first. Then whilst prepared and steady, you could try the greater superior strategies.

As the center and postural muscle tissues benefit power to preserve your body upright inside the proper posture, balance, stabilization, and arm moves can benefit greater recuperation.

Kneel in a right posture with the abs engaged.

Sit with proper posture with abs engaged.

When you have got interaction your abs, DO NOT squeeze your butt muscle agencies.

Currently, most of you have got already been thru remedy, or you are nevertheless receiving treatment. Either way, preserve in thoughts this ebook is full of know-how and sports activities to probable assist you in restoration. As I stated earlier on this ebook, I am not a bodily therapist. I am a health teacher who regularly works with clients who've completed their bodily remedy and do not recognize what else they may be able to do or how a good buy in addition their restoration can pass. The stroke survivor's recuperation does no longer stop at the same time as bodily treatment ends.

You may additionally additionally only be able to do a number of the sports activities sports proper here further to some of what your therapist has proven you. Do the carrying sports that you could do and might do efficaciously.

Begin with middle and postural sporting sports.

Standing on a balance pad, disc, BOSU® ball, or kneeling on BOSU® ball is a extremely good way to warmness up the middle and postural muscles. This moreover strengthens the ones muscle tissue and stimulates the primary frightened machine. It additionally enables educate the body to multitask another time and allows to rebuild unique reputation and quick response time. This builds balance and balance. These are high-quality warmth-up and sports to do for fall prevention.

If you are not able to apply balance props, begin reputation at the ground till you are secure and/or enhance.

Move the shoulders and the shoulder blades.

Get the muscle businesses and nerves deep within the spine activated by way of fame on one of the stability gadget or sitting on a ball (while prepared).

Move the shoulders/arm through the extraordinary movements (that are at the internet page on shoulder joint movements) the awesome that you can.

The shoulder joint movement exercise also can be completed, sitting, or standing with or without the stableness gear. Always be in a proper posture whilst exercise. Safety First!

With the exercising above, clearly popularity on in which the palms and arms are in location. Try to manipulate the peak of every arms, making the reason to maintain the hands meeting inside the center of your body and staying at the same top as you gently and slowly skip your arm to the issue and convey it back slowly with control.

Using bands may be a extraordinary deliver with the proper posture and positing. In the following photographs, I am demonstrating my bodily sports activities the use of the Anchor Point Training® Band. These bands moreover encompass a neuro address. This address permits stimulate nerves at the same time as doing the workout. I actually have found they artwork fabulously with stroke survivors.

Chapter 7: Exercises And Tips

Here are a few critical carrying sports that I definitely have located to be crucial to regaining stability, strength, and balance for constant movement. Depending on the customer, I may also additionally have them start through way of the use of sitting on a Swiss ball, reputation at the steadiness disc, or I may additionally have them start through reputation at the BOSU® ball. In all times, particularly within the beginning, I sincerely have the consumer preserve directly to a ballet barre or the squat rack bar, notwithstanding the truth that I am within the fitness studio. If you are trying those at home, make sure to have a secure object to keep onto.

In every reputation exercise:

Engage your abs. Imagine you're zipping up a zipper to vicinity on a comfortable girdle.

Be aware about your frame's region in region from head to toe.

Be aware about feet placement. Feel them lightly anchored anyplace you're reputation. Try to maintain toes frivolously placed; do now not permit them to roll out to the perimeters.

Stand up tall, stack the shoulders over the hips, and bear in mind you are lengthening your spine to the sky.

Imagine your body weight is lifting as your toes maintain the experience of being anchored within the ground.

For safety, at the same time as needed, maintain onto a bar or regular object, which permits you to maintain an superb posture.

Hold on enough to be safe, however do no longer end up so stiff which you do not experience the balancing task of the disc or BOSU® ball.

If you're sitting on the stableness (Swiss) ball, anchored as described above, keep the knees over the ankles and sit up tall collectively together with your shoulders over your hips.

Follow the instructions and guidelines listed with each of the subsequent bodily games.

Safety First!

Sitting on a chair and/or

sitting on a stability (Swiss) ball

Begin this exercise sitting on a chair or a bench of the appropriate pinnacle.

Directions listed right right here exercise to sitting on chair, bench, or ball.

Safety First!

When stability is more potent, and it's miles solid for you, it may be performed on the stability ball.

Be positive the ball is agency.

Be remarkable the ball or chair is the proper peak for you. Your hips must be degree collectively together with your knees. Do no longer sit down on a moderate ball or on a ball wherein your hips are below your knees.

Sit at the ball or chair in order that your lower legs are as near the ball as they will be without touching it.

Keep your knees immediately over your ankles. This method your shin bone could be in a immediately line from the ankle to the knee. Think of table legs coming immediately out of the desk joint, which allows the table leg to be placed straight away up and down.

Do now not allow your knees fall in or fall out, and do not squeeze your legs collectively.

Anchor your ft into the ground.

Engage your pelvic ground (if possible) with out squeezing your butt muscle agencies (glutes).

Engage your abs like you are putting on a cushty girdle.

Stack your shoulders over the hips.

In the start, a survivor may additionally moreover revel in that there are too many things to don't forget. That is ok; it's miles ordinary. Keep focusing from head to toe. This will help the body and thoughts regain better conversation consciously, in order to help rebuild the conversation subconsciously as you are making more potent the muscle tissue on your spine and middle.

A survivor's stroke-affected leg may also additionally fall out to the thing, and they will not be able to maintain a ball amongst their legs without assist from their hand or a professional. I want to have the survivor sit in a chair near a wall. I then place a ball a few of the wall and the affected leg. Then they'll be capable of use a few different ball some of the knees to do the exercising the exceptional they may.

In the previous snap shots, you may see that he's sitting collectively along along with his top frame in a twist, and the left foot is grew to become out. Your frame can also furthermore want to do that routinely however art work on preserving the proper positions with the toes and posture as in the preceding photograph with me illustrating the right setup.

Reminders and suggestions.

Remember at the same time as a foot appears, it turns the leg out as much as the hip and pelvic. This leaves the hips, pelvic, and resolution in an choppy characteristic. You want to assemble the frame evenly, no longer unevenly.

Remember, research display that after the frame is in proper posture, all the structures paintings higher.

Do the ones wearing activities in a chair in advance than you enhance to a ball.

Sitting on a chair or a Stability (Swiss) Ball - Adductor/Abductor Exercise

Use a Bender® ball or a small mild Pilates ball and gently squeeze the diverse knees/internal thighs. This may be completed along with your toes flat at the ground and tiptoes.

Set up in right posture and positioning at the ball or chair.

Place the ball among your knees or inner thighs, anywhere it feels snug for you.

Recheck your role and posture and enjoy as in case you are setting on that girdle and lengthen the spine up tall with the abs engaged.

Gently, however firmly squeeze the ball among your knees (inner thighs) with manage, then release with manage. Repeat this movement for 10 to twenty reps. Be positive to apply the same pace at some point of the exercising. (Try NOT to squeeze the ball after which short "snap" the discharge.) Work your self up to a few units of 20 reps. (This amount adjustments and varies in line with person). When I am walking with a customer, we communicate and determine together the big variety that works for them based completely at the electricity and potential of the client.

DO NOT squeeze the butt (glutes) at the equal time as performing this workout. For maximum human beings, this takes awareness.

As with any wearing sports, in case your lower again, hip, or knee joints damage on the same time as doing this exercise, first recheck your form, and if that doesn't restoration it, STOP the workout!

It is by no means a extremely good idea to harm one vicinity of the body to bolster each other. Proper physical sports that works for the entire body, while retaining off injuries, is crucial.

As you decorate with this workout, and it's far secure as a way to do, you could area a balance pad or balance disc beneath your ft as you're taking a seat in the chair or the ball. This will supply extra of a assignment in stability, balance, spatial hobby, proprioception, and neutrally.

Standing on the Balance

Pad and Balance Disc

If you're the usage of a stability disc, the disc have to no longer be too flimsy. I surely have placed that the CanDo® emblem, 35cm/thirteen inches, is a exceptional one to apply. I have located mine on Amazon.

Engage your abs. Imagine you are zipping up a zip to region on a comfortable girdle earlier than even stepping onto the steadiness disc. Re-have interaction your abs after you are popularity on the balance disc.

Be aware about the body's vicinity in region from head to toe.

Be aware about feet placement. Feel them calmly anchored in which you're fame. Try to preserve your ft frivolously positioned; do no longer allow them to roll out to the rims.

Stand up tall, stack your shoulders up over your hips, and remember you are accomplishing the top of your head to the sky.

Imagine your frame weight is lifting as your toes keep the texture of being anchored to the ground.

Hold onto a bar or consistent item so you can maintain an extremely good posture, however do now not preserve the frame so stiff that you do now not experience the balancing task of the disc.

Depending on each survivor's balance power or worrying situations, one must typically start at their very own degree.

Beginning with a stability pad before the disc is also recommended and often desired.

The above instructions are the same that comply with while recognition on the ground, a disc, a pad, or the BOSU ball®.

Standing on the BOSU® Ball

You ought to have the BOSU® ball inflated to its proper firmness. Usually, if you turn the BOSU® ball over in order that the platform is coping with up and diploma the gap from the floor to the top of the platform, it ought to be about nine to ten inches off the floor. I truly have discovered that BOSU® balls can variety a piece in duration. A flatter ball DOES NOT MEAN IT'S A BETTER CHALLENGE. That isn't always how it works; it is not the era at the back of this piece of machine.

Engage your abs. Imagine you're zipping up a zip to position on a snug girdle earlier than even stepping up from the floor. Re-engage your abs whilst you are repute at the BOSU® ball.

Be aware of your frame's vicinity in region from head to toe.

Be aware of ft placement. Feel them frivolously anchored to in that you are popularity. Try to keep your toes lightly located and do now not permit them to roll out to the perimeters.

Stand up tall, stack your shoulders up over your hips and don't forget you're reaching the pinnacle of your head to the sky.

Imagine that your body weight is lifting as your feet keep the feel of being anchored.

Hold onto a bar or strong item so you can preserve pinnacle posture, but do no longer hold the frame so stiff which you do now not feel the balancing undertaking of the BOSU® ball.

Depending in your character balance strength or demanding situations, you have to constantly start at your very personal degree.

Reminders and recommendations.

Practice recognition at the floor with the bar first, until you're strong enough and solid sufficient to try it on an volatile ground.

To start, take a step out, then deliver the feet collectively, then step to the side another time.

Safety first!

When you are extra advanced, you can placed an exercising band on the bar to characteristic more strengthening and balance. I like to apply the Anchorpoint Training Bands, as visible inside the next images.

I especially like the use of the Anchorpoint Training Bands with the unique neuro handles.

Taking side steps on the same time as preserving onto a band as I am doing inside the pix works stability, stabilization, posture, center, spatial recognition, and proprioception further to schooling the steps in movement.

Taking Steps to the Side

Hold the bar for stability and protection.

Try now not to stressful the fingers, shoulders, and neck whilst maintaining onto the bar.

Stand tall.

Abs engaged.

Relax shoulders. Keep the shoulders down a long way from your ears.

Try to maintain the foot that appears directed ahead, like inside the illustrations.

Start with feet together, then the first step foot out, then deliver the opposite foot to it.

Take steps sideways in every tips the complete period of your bar.

Try to keep the feet pointing beforehand through the movements.

This workout will assist restore foot drop, drag, and hyperextended knee if you are very conscious and targeted on every step.

Try not to permit the foot drag to your steps.

Lift each foot consciously off the floor even as taking every step.

Do this along the bar as many steps as you can take (relying on the duration of your bar), then move again the opposite course.

Stay upright in right balance.

Try no longer to pull each foot.

Stay aware about what every toes are doing in every step. This is spatial recognition. You also are looking to regain spatial recognition of in which your ft are in space. This is a part of fall prevention schooling.

Try not to permit your palms pull you inside the side steps. Holding on to the bar is supposed to hold you stable and balanced so that you can artwork to your ft' steps and posture.

Taking side steps at the equal time as being targeted on each placement does a few topics.

1.   This makes one recognition on in which the toes are in movement.

2.   While taking steps, purposely putting the foot inside the right role (not grew to become out) continues the hips and the muscle tissue above the foot in their accurate positions, which strengthens them in an appropriate positions for preserving the foot on top of things unconsciously once more.

three. If you're able, strive not to permit the foot drag, through purposely lifting the foot off the ground for each step.

4.   This is one shape of "information where your toes are in location," moreover called spatial popularity and a part of proprioception.

If you are risky and unsure of your balance and coordination, have someone constantly with you while you do your taking walks and stepping wearing sports. Holding onto the bar and taking facet steps back and forth across the length of the bar helps the hip and leg abductor and adductor muscle agencies in addition to schooling and regaining the relationship to the spatial recognition of in which your toes are in location.

Practicing Walking

If you are not able to practice a treadmill to exercise your strolling on, use the bar.

When practising walking, ALWAYS use the bar in case you are unstable, and you've were given balance and stabilization stressful conditions nevertheless. Stand sideways close to the bar and hold on at the side of your more potent side's hand. Always check your posture, stand tall, and workout your strolling in super form. Remember to move your very very own pace and the stroke-affected pace you need to be at to be secure.

If you may, try to hold the foot from dragging and/or turning out on the identical time as you are taking your steps, with the beneficial resource of purposely lifting the foot off the floor for every step.

Walking Backward and

Backward Movements

Walking backward may want to likely seem stupid, however it is good for you physical and mentally. We take steps backward regularly in our each day activities. Walking backward enhances the enjoy of body focus. It increases frame coordination and motion of the frame in space. Research has shown on foot backward improves forward taking walks abilties. It is said to sharpen your questioning abilties, decorate cognitive manage, and positioned the senses into overdrive. This motion additionally places less pressure on and requires lots much less variety of movement from the knee joints.

Everyone wishes to have recognition as to in which the "body is in place." Athletes need to exercise and educate with centered reputation on wherein their frame is in place for characteristic, velocity, and agility. They benefit better balance, pace, and faster response time, which might be specially essential abilities for sports activities activities sports, especially speedy-transferring sports. Stroke survivors need to regain the ones abilities for everyday life moves and regain quick reactions. Some examples: within the occasion that they pressure; moving quick to the brake pedal at the same time as preferred; shifting their foot speedy to keep away from tripping and falling or warding off losing an object on the floor.

I without a doubt have heard jogging footwear advocate having a client stroll backward on a treadmill to assist boom attention and foot placement, however I am NOT cushty with that. I experience strolling backward on a treadmill belt IS UNSAFE. I recommend having a survivor do it on the floor inside the front of a reflect that will see and experience the foot placements. If you do not like searching in the mirror, watch your toes and taking walks gait within the replicate.

REMEMBER TO USE A BAR.

Practice taking walks beforehand every day. Be superb you are not by myself or have a professional with you in case you are unstable. BE stable!

Only practice taking walks backward if you could as it should be gain this.

Walk alongside the bar to preserve onto it.

If you do no longer have control of putting each foot precisely in which you need it whilst you step, walking backward will now not be regular to do. Safety First!

After doing the preceding sports activities sports for some time, the capability to walk backward also can experience secure again.

If you're unstable and uncertain of your balance and coordination, have a person commonly with you even as you do your taking walks and stepping bodily activities.

If you're using a walker, DO NOT DO THE WALKING BACKWARDS EXERCISE.

Stepping on and stale the BOSU® ball

USE A BAR FOR SAFETY IF NEEDED!

Engage your center as described in Exercise 1 or for the stableness disc in advance than even stepping onto the dome of the BOSU® ball.

Spend a few minutes status and balancing.

When you're organized to step up and down, remind yourself to stay targeted and aware of every foot's placement as you step up and step down.

Come to an entire stability as quickly as each toes are at the dome. Stand up tall, stacking your shoulders over your hips.

When you feel balanced, stay targeted, and then step once more to the floor.

Once you come back to a whole balance on the ground, rise up tall, stacking your shoulders over your hips. Then step lower back onto the dome.

If possible, begin thru stepping up with the proper foot and stepping down with the right foot. Do this 5 times; then switch to stepping up with the left foot and stepping down with the left foot.

Work your self up to 10 on every element.

If you for my part have a foot drag, a drop project, or a few different bodily assignment or weak aspect, making this hard to do, KEEP PRACTICING. It may also additionally get less complex with time. But protection first! The extra you're repetitive with a movement, the better danger the thoughts has of making the cutting-edge pathways wanted for this sort of movement.

When stepping off to the floor, reputation on clearing the dome. The intention isn't always to permit your foot drag down the dome or hit the plastic platform. If you have got were given more bodily demanding conditions, this motion will consist of time. KEEP PRACTICING.

When finished with stepping up and down, pass lower again to in reality fame and balancing. You will find you can stability better now. If the primary few times you do now not experience this, it's going to include time. KEEP PRACTICING.

This is an specifically vital workout to help you regain stability and rebuild a strong and robust taking walks gait. It enables to rebuild an recognition of the vicinity of your feet in region in a few unspecified time within the destiny of your movement.

We take small steps stepping backwards commonly each day:

When we open a door in the route human beings.

When we technique a chair to sit down down down.

Doing laundry.

Stepping down a ladder or step.

Backing a protracted manner from the rest room or kitchen sink.

Using your ft to push your self in a chair far from a desk before you

Stand.

If you're having a hard time with the workout of walking backwards, begin with the workout of stepping up and down at the BOSU® ball first, and/or consist of it in your exercise software application earlier than you work on strolling backward.

Reminders and guidelines.

Remember, the mind sends a message to the deep middle muscle tissue to stabilize the body before movement.

If you are unable to step on the same old BOSU® ball, use a infant-length BOSU® ball if you are succesful. The purchaser on this picture modified into satisfactory 4 toes eleven.

You also can use a container or a step that is secure to apply as an exercising prop for stepping up and down, as mounted in the next pictures.

Two precise carrying sports are being confirmed in the ones pix.

The 1st Picture is demonstrating easy stepping up and down.

The 2nd photograph is extra superior. This is stepping up and lifting the leg immoderate, then stepping backtrack.

The first workout is beginning for re-getting to know stepping up on steps. The use of the BOSU® ball is more superior.

In all of the sporting events for stepping up and down, use the bar for protection.

Engage your abs and stand in proper posture.

Step completely onto a few thing you are stepping on. Do no longer allow a part of your toes preserve off the prop you're using.

If you're the usage of the BOSU® ball, step completely onto the middle of the ball. See feet positions at the same time as reputation on BOSU® ball on this ebook.

Step every toes sincerely directly to the step, stability pad, or BOSU® ball.

Once you have got each toes on your stepping prop, stand tall and be in real posture in advance than you step backtrack off the prop.

As you step off, attention on clearing the prop that you are using.

Once every ft are at the ground, stand tall and get in an tremendous posture, in advance than stepping lower back up another time.

This may take time and masses of practice. Remember that you also are re-training spatial attention of in which your toes are in area as you go together with the drift again to step down similarly to at the same time as you step up.

Only do that workout and any exercise if you are regular.

Remember Safety First!

In time this could help you be more secure taking stairs.

Squats Holding without delay to a Bar

This exercise can be completed fame on the ground or reputation on a stability pad or the BOSU® ball.

Reminders and recommendations.

It is a clever idea to exercise reputation at the floor first.

When you're prepared, workout on the stability pad.

Then while geared up beef up to the use of the stability disc and BOSU® ball.

Safety First!

This exercising is extra advanced, and some survivors can try this, and others might not. Remember to paintings at your very very very own tempo and functionality.

Begin through doing this exercising along with your ft at the floor first. Be certain you may preserve the proper alignment correctly earlier than you begin acting this at the dome of the BOSU® ball. You also can try this repute on a balance pad. When you're stronger, you may do squats with the BOSU® ball. Safety First!

While going through the bar, flippantly keep immediately to the bar in conjunction with your arms, genuinely so your body is focused amongst your fingers.

Engage your middle and recognition. Hold the frame in proper shape from head to toe, such as the shoulders.

Sit again as in case you are going to sit down down in a chair, then boom yourself decrease lower returned up.

Try to use your legs and glutes to do the movement. Do not permit the hands to do all of the artwork.

Do now not drop the hips below the knees.

If this bothers your knees, take a look at your shape. If it though bothers your knees, do now not do the exercising.

If you are doing this fame at the ground, pull yourself as a great deal as a wonderful posture among each squat.

If you are doing this at the BOSU® ball, pull your self up to perfect posture and balance your self right away up and down in right shape among each squat.

Maintain manage and recognition at some point of each motion.

In each squat, ensure each ft are parallel just so your hips and pelvis are moving frivolously thru each factors at some stage in every rep.

If you are using the BOSU® ball, do approximately eight-10 squats; then spend a few minutes balancing at the BOSU® ball. When you're more potent, artwork up to three units of 10 squats, balancing in amongst.

Work your way as a lot because the squatting. Depending on anybody's functionality, a survivor won't feel steady to do the squats in the first few weeks or maybe months.

Safety First!

Reminders and hints.

Extra Tip: Often, if a survivor locations a bean bag on their head, it facilitates with posture.

This enables join the feeling to wherein the top is in area and allows extend the pinnacle torso proper into a better posture.

Battling Ropes

Battling ropes, moreover known as battle ropes, are a top notch tool for stroke survivors and those with balance and neurological traumatic situations. They work properly for neurorehabilitation for stroke, brain accidents, cardiac rehab patients and are notable for age-associated illness. Battle ropes have a low chance of damage and are non-effect weight resistance. There is a 2-vector strain direction created whilst using the warfare ropes. This approach that one course of strain is pulling some distance from the character even as a downward strain from the pull of gravity from the weight of the ropes. This motives multiple contractions of various muscle businesses at the identical time. As this is taking region, the ropes task the dynamic balance and stabilization at the same time as the usage of them. They are being used more and more for rehabilitation and corrective sports activities. They help with asymmetrical stabilization issues. Depending on the healing level in a stroke survivor, one also can most effective use one rope at a time or ropes at a time. There are considered one of a kind wave styles to apply with the ropes that create pace and disturbing situations the center muscle organizations in particular patterns.

Individuals can use ropes in wheelchairs and walkers. They can be seated in their wheelchairs or on a chair that is the proper pinnacle for his or her pinnacle and hip degree. They can be used sitting on a ball, standing at the floor, and standing and sitting on the BOSU® ball, squatting, lunging, kneeling, and extra. I took a Battling Rope Coach Certification course with NESTA to higher my understanding the usage of the ropes with customers. There is thousands more to combating ropes then I am mentioning in this e-book.

There are masses of bodily video games that can be carried out with them. The ropes are available unique lengths, diameters, and weights.

Here are a few basic suggestions. Understand the cause of the most effective-of-a-kind hand grips. Maintain proper posture. Have the shoulder girdles set in proper alignment.

A survivor may be able to use each ropes proper away, or they will use a single rope. It will depend upon the individual demanding conditions they may be working through. The manner the fingers grip the battle ropes make a distinction. If an character has an arm so as to not paintings nicely with the ropes however, use a single rope with the double hand grip. If viable, carry out the sports activities in a single feature; then rotate the palms, so the alternative hand is on pinnacle and perform the bodily games again. The more potent arm, of direction, is probably on pinnacle of things, but the different arm will study in motion and take part in the workout as well, however with guidance from the opportunity hand. I recommend acting making waves with the battle ropes and the tsunamis. These can be completed reputation or kneeling at the floor, sitting in a chair, wheelchair, curler walker, Swiss ball, status, and sitting at the BOSU® ball.

Different Hand Grips May Be Used While Using Battle Ropes.

Combining war ropes with a few Pilates ab bodily sports is likewise a amazing supply if the survivor's hands or shoulders can do it. In this exercise, the ropes are wrapped securely spherical a pole. This purchaser is maintaining the shoulders in region, and her abs are engaged as she slowly lifts one leg and lowers it backpedal with manage at the same time as shifting on the same pace every hints. She then rotates the right and the left leg with control. Combining this exercise with the ropes is a more superior way of strengthening the middle, palms, and shoulder stabilization. These are 30-pound, 30-foot ropes. They are available in specific lengths, diameters, and weights.

The ropes are generally a laugh for the clients. Many sports activities can be carried out with them. It is a few element they should buy and use at home as quickly as they are able to use them efficiently and recognize the manner to keep away from harm using them on their non-public. They are great for neuro, aerobic, and entire-frame sports.

Here are a few Exercises

for the glutes and legs.

If you're no longer capable of visit the ground thoroughly or hold in these positions, do not do the floor physical video video games. Do the repute one maintaining onto a bar.

This first instance is a status exercising that physical video games the glutes and some hip rotation muscle agencies.

Stand on the bar, as seen in the instance.

Stand tall, precise posture, and interact your abs and your glutes engaged.

Turn one foot barely on an attitude, as seen in the instance.

Lift and decrease the leg, as visible inner the instance.

Lift the leg by using major with the glutes, NOT your foot.

This ought to be a managed movement. Lifting the leg and lowering the leg with control. Control the motion in every instructions. It is NOT a kicking up the leg and drops the leg exercise. Focus on lifting and decreasing the leg.

As you try to control the movements, it is able to be hard. This isn't unusual.

This repute exercising can be included with the ground exercising for folks that can do each.

It is k to honestly do this status exercising if you are not able to visit the ground. Remember, Safety First!

Reminders and suggestions.

In time with exercising, repetitiveness, and being steady with movements, the frame has a danger to comprehend exercising moves and assemble the today's pathways desired. As you gain yet again actions in sports activities, this transfers over to normal existence actions and sports.

Don't surrender!

I name the subsequent exercising the Bent Leg Lift. Proper positioning is essential. Think of your frame as a desk, and all 4 table legs need to return decrease back straight away down out of the corners of the tabletop. In this option, your knees want to be beneath your hips and the elbows beneath your shoulders, as verified inside the following pix with the checkmark. I understand a few stroke survivors can do floor carrying sports, and others can't. Only do the sports which could pertain to you at every step in your improvement.

Chapter 8: Understanding Stroke

A stroke, which takes vicinity whilst blood deliver to part of your thoughts is compromised, is the mind's equal of a coronary coronary heart attack. This may get up even as blood arteries are obstructed or because of mind bleeding. Strokes are a essential clinical emergency that calls for rapid care if the affected man or woman is to avoid severe damage or lack of life.

A STROKE IS WHAT?

A stroke is a doubtlessly lethal condition that takes place even as there is inadequate blood float to a exceptional region of your mind. A blocked artery or cerebral bleeding are the maximum not unusual reasons of this. The thoughts cells there start to degenerate from a loss of oxygen without a regular go along with the go together with the glide of blood.

Important: Because a stroke is a probably deadly emergency situation, each 2d counts. Call 911 (or the community emergency services sizeable variety) proper away in case you or a member of your enterprise well-knownshows symptoms of a stroke. Your possibilities of improving without handicap growth with the charge of treatment for stroke.

Keep in mind to BE FAST at the equal time as figuring out stroke symptoms and signs and symptoms:

B. A sudden loss of equilibrium need to be expected.

E. Be searching for an sudden lack of imaginative and prescient in a unmarried or each eyes. Are they seeing topics two times?

F. You have to ask them to smile. An indication of muscle weak point or paralysis is a slump on one or both in their facets of the face.

A. Muscle dropping on one facet is a commonplace symptom of stroke. Request that they enhance their arms. If they will be susceptible on one issue (and were now not in advance than), one arm will stay higher while the opportunity sags and drops beneath.

S. A individual's capability to speak is often misplaced after a stroke. They can slur their terms or have problems finding the proper ones.

T. Don't eliminate to are looking for help because of the reality time is critical! If the least bit viable, undergo in thoughts searching at a clock or your watch to keep in mind the onset of signs and symptoms. The great treatment options for you will be determined via the healthcare expert if you allow them to recognise at the equal time as your signs and signs first appeared.

WHO IS IT INTENDED FOR?

From babies to adults, absolutely everyone could have a stroke, regardless of the reality that some humans are more at hazard than others. About -thirds of strokes rise up in oldsters over the age of sixty five, making them greater well-known in later lifestyles.

Additional scientific problems that improve the danger of stroke include immoderate blood strain (excessive blood strain), hyperlipidaemia (immoderate ldl ldl cholesterol), type 2 diabetes, and a history of stroke, coronary coronary heart attack, or abnormal heartbeats like atrial disturbing inflammation.

HOW FREQUENT ARE STROKES?

A lot of humans get strokes. Strokes are the second one major cause of death inside the whole global. Stroke is the sixth best purpose of mortality in the US. Worldwide, strokes are one of the vital reasons of disability.

HOW MAY HAVING A STROKE EFFECT MY BODY?

The equal way a coronary coronary heart assault influences your coronary heart, strokes have an effect in your brain. A part of your thoughts loses blood go along with the float inside the direction of a stroke, preventing that location from receiving oxygen. The mind cells become oxygen-starved with out oxygen and forestall functioning normally.

Your thoughts cells will expire inside the occasion that they lack oxygen for an prolonged time period. You can lose the powers that place at the beginning managed if sufficient thoughts cells in that vicinity die, causing everlasting damage. However, growing blood go with the flow could probable prevent that kind of harm from occurring or at least reduce its severity. Time is therefore essential in the stroke remedy manner.

WHAT VARIETIES OF STROKE EXIST?

Haemorrhage and ischemia are the 2 most important reasons of strokes.

SCHIZOPHRENIC STROKE

When cells do not accumulate sufficient blood glide to offer them with oxygen, it is known as ischemia (advised "iss-key-me-uh"). Usually, some component obstructs a blood vessel to your mind, preventing the go with the flow of blood. About 80% of all strokes are ischemic in nature, making them the most common type.

Most ischemic strokes arise in one of the following methods:

The development of a thrombus on your mind.

An embolism is the discharge of a bit of a blood clot that has developed a few area else for your frame, which travels via your blood vessels and resorts for your mind.

Small vessel blockage (lacunar stroke), that could occur as a result of untreated, chronically excessive blood stress (high blood pressure), hyperlipidaemia (high ldl cholesterol), or Type 2 diabetes.

Unknown reasons (those strokes are cryptogenic; "cryptogenic" way "hidden foundation").

stroke with haemorrhage

Blood clots shape inner or spherical your mind because of haemorrhagic strokes (said "hem-or-aj-ick"). There are viable conditions for this:

Internal bleeding (intracerebral bleeding). This takes location at the same time as a blood vessel indoors your brain bursts or tears, creating bleeding that exerts stress on the close by mind tissue.

Bleeding into your mind's subarachnoid space, that is the place among your thoughts and its protecting shielding. Your mind is encased in a skinny layer of tissue known as the arachnoid membrane, which has a pattern similar to a spiderweb. The subarachnoid location (the prefix "sub" manner "under") is the place of your mind that it occupies. A subarachnoid haemorrhage, which includes bleeding into the subarachnoid region and placing strain at the mind tissue underneath, can be delivered on with the beneficial resource of harm to blood vessels that go with the flow via the arachnoid membrane.

CAUSES AND SYMPTOMS

What signs and symptoms and signs and symptoms and symptoms and signs and symptoms and signs and symptoms factor to a stroke?

The signs and signs of a stroke variety counting on the a part of the mind that is injured for the reason that one-of-a-type mind areas govern diverse capacities. A stroke that impacts the area of your thoughts referred to as Broca's, which regulates how your face and mouth muscular tissues art work to talk, is an instance of this. This is why some individuals who get a stroke conflict to talk or slur their phrases.

stroke signs and symptoms may additionally encompass one or more of the subsequent:

Paralysis or susceptible element on one facet.

Aphasia (hassle speakme or loss of speech).

Speaking with a slur or confusion (dysarthria).

Dyscontrol of your facial muscle groups on one element.

The sudden loss of one or greater of the senses (listening to, tasting, smelling, or touching), each absolutely or in part.

Double or distorted eyesight (diplopia).

Ataxia, a lack of coordination or clumsiness.

Unsteadiness or vertigo.

Vomiting and diarrhoea.

A stiff neck.

Alterations in person and emotional instability.

Fear or uncertainty.

Convulsions.

Amnesia, or reminiscence loss.

Migraines (usually excessive and sudden).

Passing away or becoming subconscious.

Coma.

Transient ischemic assault (TIA)

Similar to a stroke, a brief ischemic assault (TIA), additionally called a "mini-stroke," has handiest short-time period results. These are usually early caution symptoms that a person is in grave chance of having a stroke quick. A TIA victim desires emergency hospital therapy as soon as viable due to this.

WHAT TRIGGERS A STROKE?

There are severa motives why ischemic and haemorrhagic strokes may additionally appear. Ischemic strokes are typically delivered on thru blood clots. These have to appear for numerous motives, which incorporates:

Arterial stenosis.

Clotting troubles.

Atrial fibrillation, mainly if sleep apnea is at blame.

Cardiovascular sicknesses, on the facet of ventricular or atrial septal defects.

Microvascular ischemic illness, which could result in a blockage of the tiniest blood vessels inside the brain.

A amount of things can contribute to hemorrhagic strokes, at the side of: High blood strain, in particular whilst it is chronic, in particular excessive, or each.

Brain aneurysms can every now and then motive hemorrhagic strokes.

Brain tumours, in particular cancerous ones.

Disorders that harm your thoughts's blood arteries or have unusual results on them, together with moyamoya sickness.

equal conditions

Numerous different illnesses and factors can probably boom or lower one's probability of getting a stroke. These encompass: Alcohol abuse troubles.

High blood stress (immoderate blood pressure can harm blood vessels, which will increase the hazard of stroke and influences all types of strokes, now not truely hemorrhagic ones).

Hyperlipidaemia, or excessive ldl ldl cholesterol.

Migraine complications (they could have symptoms and signs and symptoms just like a stroke, and people who revel in auras, specially, have a higher danger of getting a stroke in a few unspecified time in the future in their lives).

Type 2 diabetes (T2D).

Other tobacco use, collectively with smokeless tobacco and vaporizing.

Misuse of prescription drugs, both prescribed and over-the-counter.

Is it contagious?

Since a stroke isn't contagious, it can't be passed from one man or woman to every other.

TESTING AND DETECTION

How exactly are strokes detected?

A neurological exam, diagnostic imaging, and extraordinary assessments can be used by a scientific expert to diagnose a stroke. During a neurological exam, you will be asked to do responsibilities or solution questions. The company may be gazing you while you complete those obligations or respond to the ones questions for telltale symptoms and signs that trace to an hassle with how a part of your mind functions.

What assessments could be achieved to set up the analysis of this condition?

The following exams are robotically finished even as a scientific expert detects a stroke:

a laptop tomography, or CT test.

Lab blood checks to, amongst wonderful matters, take a look at for infections or coronary heart harm, show blood sugar levels and clotting functionality, and decide the condition of the kidneys and liver.

An electrocardiogram to rule out any ability heart issues (additionally referred to as an ECG or EKG).

Magnetic resonance imaging (MRI) scans.

Despite being a splendid deal less not unusual, electroencephalograms (EEGs) can rule out seizures or different associated troubles.

PREVENTION

How can I absolutely save you or lessen my danger of getting a stroke?

There are numerous subjects you could take to reduce your hazard of getting a stroke. Even at the same time as you cannot prevent a stroke, you may decrease your risk. You can have a look at those instructions:

Modify your manner of lifestyles. Eating a balanced weight-reduction plan and exercise often can enhance your fitness. Another important thing is getting the requisite seven to 8 hours of sleep every night time time.

Refrain from making lousy life-style options and, if required, alternate your behaviour. If you smoke, use tobacco merchandise, together with vaping, use enjoyment capsules or abuse prescription prescriptions, abuse alcohol, use unlawful capsules, or smoke, you face an progressed chance of having a stroke. It's essential to finish them or in no way begin them. If you experience any of these, it's far critical that you communicate collectively in conjunction with your scientific physician. With the help of your provider, who can provide you records and belongings, you can adjust your way of life to save you sporting out the ones behaviours.

Attend for your risk elements and health difficulties. Obesity, strange cardiac rhythms, sleep apnea, excessive blood pressure, Type 2 diabetes, or high ldl cholesterol are only some of the ailments that can boom your danger of having an ischemic stroke. If you have had been given one or extra of these issues, it is critical which you take movement to manipulate your signs and symptoms and symptoms and symptoms, specially with the useful resource of taking prescription drug treatments like blood thinners as prescribed thru your health practitioner. Significant stroke-related issues may be prevented in a while by means of manner of way of doing that early in life.

Visit your primary care physician as quick as a yr for a checkup or well-being appointment. Annual nicely-being tests can pick out fitness issues, including people who growth your hazard of stroke, prolonged earlier than you've got got any signs and symptoms.

Is there some thing I need to keep away from eating at the same time as having this case?

Your doctor should recommend changing your food plan when you have any shape of stroke danger that lets in you to prevent blood strain spikes. Here are few times:

Caffeinated liquids, which includes coffee, tea, tender liquids, and so on.

Foods with immoderate salt or sodium content material material fabric, which may enhance blood strain.

Saturated-fat-rich food, alongside aspect fried dishes and other such gadgets.

Alcohol or unlawful stimulants together with cocaine, amphetamines, and methamphetamine.

PROGNOSIS / OUTLOOK

What can I count on if this is my state of affairs?

What to assume in the occasion of a stroke is based upon on a number of variables, including the size and place of the stroke inside the brain. Additionally, ischemic and hemorrhagic strokes range in a few wonderful strategies.

ISCHEMIC STROKE

In famous, the damage is worse the greater excessive the ischemic stroke is. You're more likely to lose particular abilities, at the least in short, if the thoughts damage is extra immoderate. The quicker you're looking for scientific assist for stroke signs and signs and symptoms, the greater the danger that those facet results can be quick or a lot less excessive.

STROKE WITH HAEMORRHAGE

When bleeding is extra severe at some stage in those strokes, the signs and symptoms are usually worse. Hemorrhagic stroke signs and symptoms and signs commonly go with the flow worse very quickly. Severe complications, convulsions, and coma are commonplace symptoms and symptoms of hemorrhagic stroke sufferers.

A STROKE LASTS HOW LONG?

As prolonged as part of your thoughts isn't always getting enough blood, you're having a stroke. If left untreated, a stroke will persist until the mind cells inside the affected regions of your thoughts perish, leaving your mind sincerely broken.

The signs and symptoms and signs and symptoms of a stroke can remain even after you have were given obtained treatment. The majority of people need weeks or even months to get higher. Within the number one six to 18 months (roughly) following a stroke, the bulk of recuperation improvement takes area. After that, further improvement stays possible but may be greater difficult or need more time.

WHEN MAY I RETURN TO MY JOB OR STUDIES?

When you could resume your normal sports activities and time table, your healthcare practitioner is the excellent character to endorse you. But it is vital now not to over exert oneself. You danger having some different stroke or developing one among a kind troubles if you don't have enough time to get better.

WHAT IS THIS CONDITION'S PROGNOSIS?

When strokes are extreme or keep untreated for an prolonged time frame, they'll bring about dying. However, a number of variables may additionally despite the fact that have a considerable impact on the diagnosis. The vicinity of the stroke in your mind, its severity, your medical facts, and different factors are among them.

The high-quality man or woman to tell you of the outlook in your case is your healthcare scientific doctor. The information they offer may be the maximum precise and pertinent information you could find.

DETECTION AND TESTS

Exactly how are strokes identified?

A scientific expert can pick out out a stroke via manner of manner of the usage of a neurological examination, diagnostic imaging, and other trying out. You may be requested to do responsibilities or respond to questions in some unspecified time in the future of a neurological exam. The issuer will watch you as you entire those responsibilities or respond to those questions for telltale signs that thing to an problem with how part of your thoughts features.

What checks can be run to determine this example's assessment?

When a scientific expert suspects a stroke, the subsequent assessments are regularly completed:

a CT test, or laptop tomography.

Lab blood assessments to test for infections or coronary coronary heart harm, degree blood sugar ranges and clotting potential, and affirm the fitness of the kidneys and liver, among one of a kind subjects.

Electrocardiogram (additionally called an ECG or EKG) to rule out any capability coronary coronary coronary heart issues.

Scans using magnetic resonance imaging (MRI).

Electroencephalograms (EEGs), notwithstanding being plenty a whole lot much less commonplace, can rule out seizures or special related problems.

Chapter 9: Medical Treatment And Rehabilitation

HOW ARE STROKES HANDLED?

There are severa variables that have an impact on stroke treatment. What type of stroke an individual gets is the most vital problem in figuring out treatment.

Ischemic: The cause of remedy for ischemic strokes is to reestablish blood go with the flow to the factors of the thoughts. Sometimes, if this occurs brief sufficient, it's miles feasible to avoid irreparable harm or at least reduce the severity of a stroke. A catheterization technique also can be crucial for the recuperation of flow, which generally involves a class of medication called thrombolytics.

Hemorrhagic: The direction of treatment for hemorrhagic strokes varies on wherein and what shape of bleeding is gift. The first motive is regularly lowering blood strain because of the truth doing so will lessen the quantity of bleeding and save you it from growing worse.

Enhancing clotting is a exquisite method of remedy which could make the bleeding stop. When blood builds up for your brain, surgical treatment can be required to release the stress.

WHAT DRUGS OR THERAPIES ARE EMPLOYED?

Depending on the form of stroke and the way soon after the stroke the affected character receives care, unique drugs and treatments are employed. There are different lengthy-term stroke treatments available. These take location inside the days and months following emergency contend with the stroke's without delay risk.

In preferred, the amazing individual to inform you of the encouraged remedy(s) is your healthcare professional. They can adjust the facts they offer to your specific scenario based totally for your medical history, personal times, and further.

Here are a few examples of stroke treatments:

Ischemic stroke

Hemorrhagic stroke

capsules that skinny the blood (interior three to four hours).

manipulate of blood pressure.

Thrombectomy (if there hasn't been any severe thoughts damage, inside 24 hours). Any treatment that would make bleeding worse want to be stopped.

control of blood pressure. Using tablets or having surgical operation to alleviate strain inside the skull.

MEDICATION THAT THINS THE BLOOD

Within the number one three hours following the onset of stroke signs and signs and symptoms and symptoms and symptoms, thrombolytic drug remedies are a probable treatment choice (the decision is a mixture of the Greek phrases "thrombus," which means that that "clot," and "lysis," this means that "loosening/dissolving"). Existing clots are broken up through those drugs. But beyond that, they enhance the possibility of risky bleeding problems, as a end result they should simplest be used within that three-to-four-and-a-half of-hour window.

MACHINE-ASSISTED THROMBECTOMY

Mechanical thrombectomy, a catheterization operation, is an opportunity in a few conditions, in particular while thrombolytic medicinal pills are not an possibility. The most green time to have a thrombectomy is inner 24 hours after the onset of symptoms and signs because of the fact this surgery is also time-touchy. This operation includes guiding a catheter-like tool as an entire lot as the blood clot for your thoughts with the beneficial useful resource of placing it right right into a big blood vessel. Once there, the catheter includes a device that could put off the clot at its tip.

MANAGEMENT OF BLOOD PRESSURE

Because hemorrhagic strokes are generally because of immoderate blood strain, lowering blood pressure is an essential aspect of treating them. Blood strain discount reduces bleeding and lets in clotting, which permits to seal the injured blood artery.

SUPPORTING CLOTTING

Haemostasis, a way your frame uses to prevent bleeding and heal wounds, is a key component of clotting. In order to assist haemostasis, pills or blood additives that facilitate coagulation are infused. Prothrombin or clotting element infusions, vitamins K remedy, and different processes are examples. Especially for folks that take blood-thinning pills, this treatment, this is most customarily used for hemorrhagic strokes, can assist restrict bleeding.

SURGERY

Surgery may additionally additionally from time to time be required to launch strain on your mind. This is specifically actual for subarachnoid haemorrhages due to the reality they're positioned at the out of doors of your mind and are consequently plenty much less complex to get right of entry to.

numerous strategies, which include supportive recovery techniques

There are severa additional methods that a stroke is probably treated. While some of these remedies proper now beneficial useful useful resource in recovery, others resource in preventing issues. You can research extra approximately those greater remedy plans out of your healthcare expert, together with which ones they endorse and why.

TREATMENT FOR STROKE

Assistance in restoration or model to the adjustments within the mind is one of the most critical stroke remedies. That is especially right close to to helping human beings in improving abilities that that they had earlier than the stroke. For the bulk of stroke patients, rehabilitation is an essential element of recuperation. Many distinct kinds of rehabilitation are possible, which encompass:

Speech therapy: This can useful resource on your recovery of language and talking abilties similarly to your functionality to modify the muscle businesses that aid respiratory, consuming, consuming, and swallowing.

Physical therapy: This permit you to in improving or regaining the usage of your arms, palms, feet, and legs. Additionally, it is able to useful resource with balance problems, muscle weak spot, and awesome issues.

Occupational treatment: will allow you to retrain your mind so that you can keep about your normal obligations. The precise hand moves and muscle manipulate which might be stepped forward with the useful resource of this treatment are specially useful.

If you're having memory issues, cognitive remedy can be beneficial. If you discover it tough to consciousness or focus on responsibilities which you used to have the ability to finish, it is able to additionally be of help.

Depending to your scenario and times, particular remedy can be appropriate. The awesome person to inform you what forms of remedy alternatives will assist you is your healthcare professional.

TREATMENT SIDE EFFECTS/COMPLICATIONS

The unfavourable effects of stroke remedies range appreciably counting on the type of stroke, the remedy alternatives carried out, your medical heritage, and different factors. More statistics at the damaging results you may or need to count on, in addition to what you may do to manipulate or even save you them, is to be had out of your healthcare organisation.

WHAT CAN I DO TO LOOK FOR MYSELF OR CONTROL THE SYMPTOMS?

You want to in no way try to self-diagnose or self-deal with a stroke due to the fact it's miles a vital medical emergency. You need to dial 911 (or your nearby emergency services range) right away if you or a person you are with research stroke signs and symptoms and symptoms. The chance of growing irreversible thoughts damage or loss of existence from a stroke will boom the longer it waits to begin treatment.

WHEN WILL I START TO FEEL BETTER FOLLOWING TREATMENT?

After remedy, some of variables have an impact on how lengthy it's going to take if you want to get better and enjoy better. The awesome man or woman to recommend you what to anticipate and when your restoration will probable get up is your healthcare expert.

QUICK MEDICAL ATTENTION FOR A STROKE

To lessen capability thoughts damage and boom recuperation possibilities, it's miles crucial to understand the signs of a stroke and are trying to find for activate emergency medical interest. This web web page gives a comprehensive creation to emergency scientific take care of stroke, which include identifying the signs and symptoms, appearing speedy, and comprehending the available treatment alternatives.

IDENTIFYING THE SYMPTOMS

Early intervention requires an data of the symptoms and signs and symptoms of a stroke. Keep in thoughts the letters "FALT":

1. Face: Have them smile on the equal time as you look for any facial sagging on one factor.

2. Arms: Have the hassle growth every fingers as you look for any arm slackness or flow.

3. Listen carefully for slurred speech or different signs of problem speakme or statistics.

4. Time: It's important to act brief. Make an emergency name as quick as you check any of those symptoms.

RESOLVING IMMEDIATELY

It is vital to answer quick at the same time as a stroke is suspected:

First, dial emergency offerings: Call the emergency line to your kingdom (for instance, 911 in the US) and allow them to recognise that you assume you'll be having a stroke. Describe in which you're and another pertinent information.

2. Stay with the person: Stay with the injured man or woman till useful aid may be rendered. Keep them cushty and reassure them.

3. Don't Offer Meals or Medicine: Giving food or remedy thru mouth need to be avoided until medical specialists recommend in any other manner on account that aspiration in the path of a stroke is viable.

Notice the Time: The 2d the symptoms started out need to be recalled or said. For selecting the extraordinary path of treatment, this data is important.

MEDICAL EMERGENCY CARE

The following actions can be part of instant scientific remedy for a stroke:

1. Pre-health facility care is the first step: Paramedics examine the affected individual's fitness and crucial symptoms.

They may moreover want to begin administering therapy right away, which encompass starting an IV and giving oxygen.

2. Patient Arrival at the Hospital: The affected character is taken to the nearest scientific facility that could deal with them, ideally a stroke centre with specialised remedy.

The scientific group makes a short exam, evaluating the patient's neurological situation and using imaging checks like a CT or MRI to pinpoint the kind and location of the stroke.

Blood samples are accrued to degree variables such as clotting factors, blood sugar levels, and other inclinations.

Chapter 10: Physical Rehabilitation

One sort of rehabilitation is physical remedy, which aids in helping patients regain or decorate their range of motion and useful abilities. It is often applied in the aftermath of a stroke, spinal cord harm, or a few other neurological sickness. Physical therapists rent a number of strategies to help sufferers with their physical rehabilitation, along with:

Exercise: Physical rehabilitation involves exercise. Strength, mobility, and coordination are all more applicable through it.

Manual remedy: This kind of arms-on remedy can help lessen ache and improve joint mobility, muscular tone, and stiffness.

Gait schooling: This technique allows people end up extra adept at transferring through region.

Balance schooling: People who have interaction in stability schooling locate that their coordination and stability have superior.

Functional education: Functional schooling teaches humans the way to perform ADLs like dressing, bathing, and ingesting.

EXERCISE RESOURCES FOR STROKE REHABILITATION

For stroke recovery, there are a brilliant fashion of exercising programs available. The following are some of the most regular kinds of workout programs:

Exercises that growth form of movement in the joints are known as range-of-movement bodily sports.

Strengthening muscle electricity is aided via energy education activities.

Exercises that promote stability and coordination are referred to as balancing physical sports activities.

Functional wearing activities: People can learn how to perform sports of day by day dwelling (ADLs) with the assist of practical carrying events.

Depending on someone's particular necessities and goals, the advanced form of fitness habitual will range. Some human beings might also want to require a utility with a selection-of-movement improvement trouble, whilst others could need a software with a power or stability improvement thing.

MOBILITY AND BALANCE INSTRUCTION

Physical remedy for the ones who have had a stroke or every different neurological contamination need to encompass mobility and stability sports. Balance is the ability to hold one's equilibrium, at the same time as mobility is the functionality to transport round. For independent residing, every motion and balance are vital.

Mobility and stability can be superior thru diverse wearing activities and sports. Walking, Tai chi, yoga, balance drills, and useful drills are some examples of common bodily video games.

According to genuinely everybody's precise dreams and dreams, the most shape of workout or pastime will range. While a few can be capable of growth to more hard sports, some human beings also can moreover need first of all less difficult wearing events.

HELPFUL AND ADAPTIVE TECHNOLOGY

People with disabilities can be able to carry out sports activities of every day residing (ADLs) with more independence within the event that they have get proper of access to to assistive technology and adaptive system. There are many numerous kinds of assistive gadget and adaptable factors to be had, along with: wheelchairs, walkers, crutches, canes, orthotics, communication gadgets, adaptive utensils, and adaptive garments.

Based on their precise desires and competencies, every body may require a one-of-a-type form of tailor-made device or assistive technology. While a few human beings would possibly satisfactory require a sincere tool, others ought to in all likelihood require a few aspect greater hard.

MUSCLE SPASTICITY MANAGEMENT

After a stroke or specific neurological disorder, spasticity of the muscle agencies is a not unusual trouble. Increased muscular tone is a defining characteristic of spasticity, that might make it tough to move the affected muscle mass. For muscle spasticity, there are numerous treatments available, which incorporates:

Medication: There are a number of tablets that may be used to deal with muscle stiffness.

Injections: Muscles that are impacted via Botox injections can loosen up.

Physical treatment: Physical remedy can beneficial resource in restoring kind of movement and capability to the muscle corporations that have been injured.

Occupational remedy: Using suitable gear and coping mechanisms to deal with spasticity, sufferers can learn how to use occupational remedy.

According to surely anybody's unique goals and goals, the gold standard form of remedy can be selected. Effective spasticity manage for sure sufferers also can require a mixture of remedies

Chapter 11: Speech And Language Therapy

AFTER A STROKE, COMMUNICATION CAN BE DIFFICULT.

The impairment to the language centres of the thoughts after a stroke may also make it difficult for people to speak. Various problems with analyzing, writing, talking, and facts language are only a few of the techniques that those impairments can seem. A man or woman's potential to unique oneself and have interaction with others effectively can be substantially impacted by manner of communique problems.

THEORIES OF SPEECH THERAPY

Speech remedy is a particular form of remedy that pastimes to decorate the readability and manufacturing of speech. SLPs, or speech-language pathologists, are educated experts who offer speech therapy to human beings with communication troubles, which consist of the ones who've had a stroke.

Several techniques are used in speech treatment to cope with precise speech troubles. Some examples of these techniques are:

a) Articulation treatment: which pastimes to make speech sounds clearer. In order to beautify common speech intelligibility, SLPs collaborate with customers to accurate speech sound issues.

b) Oral motor bodily games: These workout workouts are designed to build up the tongue and lip muscular tissues, which is probably applied to provide speech. Coordination and control of speaking moves can be more quality with their beneficial useful resource.

c) Voice abnormalities along with hoarseness or terrible vocal projection that could expand after a stroke are addressed with strategies in voice therapy. Increasing vocal loudness, pitch, and amazing are the principle dreams of voice treatment.

d) Fluency techniques: Speech therapy can contain fluency techniques to encourage greater fluid and fluent speech for people who have stuttering or other fluency troubles after a stroke.

e) Respiratory Training: Stroke patients' breathing muscular tissues can be compromised, which affects their potential to talk. Breath control and help for speech output are every advanced by manner of respiratory education bodily sports.

According to definitely all people's specific desires and targets, precise speech remedy strategies may be hired.

WELL-BEING OF THE LANGUAGE

When a person has had language problems due to a stroke, language rehabilitation goals to beautify their language comprehension and expressive abilties. It consists of dealing with problems associated with verbal expression, written verbal exchange, and language comprehension problems.

The following are some examples of methods and sporting activities that can be applied in language rehabilitation:

Exercises for improving an person's capability for know-how spoken language are included in phase a. Following instructions, responding to inquiries, and listening to and summarizing data are only a few examples of the kinds of subjects they will include.

b) Reading and Writing Therapy: Exercises for analyzing comprehension and writing expression can be part of language rehabilitation. SLPs may additionally furthermore appoint techniques together with studying aloud, word recognition drills, and writing sports to decorate language abilities.

c) Semantic and Vocabulary Training: This concentrates on improving a person's vocabulary and comprehension of phrase meanings. There are a number of techniques that may be used, alongside facet phrase establishments, categorization wearing sports, and word retrieval drills.

Exercises to enhance sentence shape, grammar, and syntax can be blanketed in language treatment. The creation of grammatically sound and coherent sentences can be aided via using the usage of the ones carrying sports.

e) Conversational Practice: It is important for people to have conversations with others a first-rate manner to increase their conversational capabilities and emerge as greater powerful communicators in normal settings. For the motive of enhancing conversational abilties, SLPs can help feature-playing, primarily based talks, and social engagement activities.

COMMUNICATION THAT IS SUPPLEMENTAL AND ALTERNATIVE

Augmentative and possibility conversation (AAC) strategies may be used for those who've enormous speech and language deficits that hold after a stroke. The term "AAC" refers to using tools and techniques for communication that both useful resource or alternative for traditional speech.

SOME AAC TECHNIQUES ARE:

a) Picture Communication Boards: These are forums or charts containing images or symbols that stand in for superb phrases or thoughts. The images or symbols may be pointed at through the usage of humans to unique their wishes and ideas.

b) Speech-generating Tools: These virtual system synthesize speech based totally on person input. They can be pre-programmed with terms or terms, permitting customers to specific themselves with the beneficial aid of choosing from to be had opportunities.

c) Text-to-Speech Apps and Software: These tools turn written textual content into spoken language. Through using written communications which may be ultimately have a take a look at aloud, they may be used on computer structures, capsules, or cell phones with the useful resource of people.

d) Sign Language or Specific Gesture Systems: Sign language or specific gesture systems may be used to assist humans talk inside the occasion that they've problem speaking.

To study every person's communication goals and pick the satisfactory AAC techniques, SLPs art work carefully with the character and their families. To ensure the powerful software of those techniques, furthermore they provide schooling and help.

In stop, speech and language remedy permits people who've had strokes with their communique issues. Speech-language pathologists artwork to enhance language comprehension, speech manufacturing, and expressive capabilities using lots of strategies and interventions. Additional techniques for assisting human beings with massive conversation troubles embody augmentative and opportunity communication strategies. The surrender end result is to beautify verbal exchange capabilities and allow vast connection in every day life.

Chapter 12: Occupational Therapy

The cause of occupational remedy (OT), a expert branch of healthcare, is to assist human beings in acquiring, regaining, or retaining the competencies required for widespread engagement in everyday sports activities sports and independence. Enhancing every day living talents, cognitive rehabilitation, art work and vocational rehabilitation, and assistive generation for independence are a number of the vital areas in which occupational remedy plays a critical function. These subjects may be explored in this essay.

IMPROVE DAILY LIVING SKILLS

Enhancing someone's functionality to perform regular activities independently is sincerely one of occupational treatment's most crucial objectives. Activities like bathing, apparel, grooming, getting prepared food, and doing chores across the residence may moreover fall beneath this elegance. To red meat up a person's abilties and help them deal with any bodily, cognitive, or emotional problems they may stumble upon, occupational therapists affirm their useful capabilities and create remedies which can be especially tailored to them. Techniques for promoting independence may moreover encompass advising supportive gadgets or device, offering training in adaptive strategies, and converting the surroundings.

BRAIN REHABILITATION

The motive of cognitive rehabilitation is to decorate cognitive capabilities like memory, hobby, hassle-fixing, and executive abilities. People who've suffered from cognitive impairments due to illnesses like stroke, annoying mind harm, or neurodegenerative issues are closely labored with thru occupational therapists. For the purpose of enhancing cognitive feature, they use masses of evidence-based totally completely interventions, which encompass cognitive retraining bodily video games, compensatory strategies, and environmental modifications.

The remaining aim is to beautify a person's capability to partake in ordinary duties like budgeting, adhering to a time table, or interacting with others.

VOCATIONAL REHABILITATION AND EMPLOYMENT

After an harm, contamination, or handicap, occupational therapists are important in supporting patients in getting decrease back to work or taking detail in enjoyable vocational sports activities sports. They determine suitable paintings settings and employment assignments with the resource of evaluating the individual's practical skills, pastimes, and goals at the facet of employers or vocational rehabilitation experts. Occupational therapists can offer interventions such artwork readiness education, ergonomic opinions, place of business modifications, and recommendation on adaptive machine. In order to enhance common art work traditional overall performance and interest delight, further they offer advice on a way to create coping mechanisms and manipulate stress.

FOR INDEPENDENCE: ASSISTING TECHNOLOGY

The term "assistive generation" refers to tools, tool, and generation that help human beings adapt for their practical boundaries and foster independence. Occupational therapists are licensed to assess patients' needs and advocate suitable assistive era answers. Mobility aids (which consist of wheelchairs or walkers), adaptive kitchenware, verbal exchange system, domestic automation structures, or pc software program software may additionally moreover all fall below this class. To make certain that human beings can efficaciously use assistive generation and include it into their normal lives, occupational therapists offer schooling, assistance, and on-going monitoring. This permits humans to complete obligations and take part in sports activities that they'll in any other case find difficult.

Chapter 13: Psychological And Emotional Recovery

The entire fitness and rehabilitation of these who have had a stroke is based upon closely on mental and emotional restoration. The outcomes of a stroke go with the flow past bodily barriers and frequently bring about emotional issues such publish-stroke emotions, melancholy, and anxiety, in addition to a name for to enlarge resilience and emotional properly-being. This article will communicate a number of critical components of mental and emotional recovery after a stroke, together with managing put up-stroke emotions, managing melancholy and tension, fostering emotional properly-being, and the importance of supportive treatment plans and counselling. It may additionally speak a way to deal with submit-stroke feelings.

MANAGING THE AFTER-STROKE EMOTIONS

A stroke can be a painful and lifestyles-changing incidence that often reasons a substantial kind of emotions, together with sadness, annoyance, rage, and grief. In order to assist people in managing those post-stroke emotions, occupational therapists, psychologists, and certainly one of a kind healthcare professionals collaborate with them. Among the feasible techniques are teaching humans approximately common emotional reactions to stroke, giving them adaptive coping skills, establishing assist agencies, and encouraging open communication with own family and caregivers. Individuals can higher adapt to their new situation and take part of their rehabilitation adventure through addressing those emotions.

MANAGING ANXIETY AND DEPRESSION

Common mental troubles that could growth after a stroke embody anxiety and despair. Assessing and treating those troubles require the assist of medical professionals, which includes psychiatrists and psychologists. Therapy, which include cognitive-behavioural remedy (CBT), which aids sufferers in spotting and converting unfavorable perception styles and behaviours, is one feasible form of remedy. In a few conditions, medicinal drug manage also can be taken into consideration. A smoother recovery manner can be accomplished with the aid of treating melancholy and anxiety, boosting emotional properly-being, and tasty in amusing sports activities. Additionally, way of life adjustments, social help, and involvement in enjoyable sports are crucial additives.

RESILIENCE AND EMOTIONAL WELL-BEING BUILDING

Individuals improving from a stroke have to boom their emotional stability and resilience. To offer individualized interventions that decorate emotional resilience, occupational therapists, psychologists, and counsellors artwork collectively. These answers could probable involve making capacity goals, gaining knowledge of the manner to clear up issues, workout strain-discount strategies, and inspiring encouraging self-speak. Creating a guide gadget and taking element in emotional nicely-being-selling hobbies, socializing, and rest carrying occasions also are essential in fostering resilience and wellknown intellectual fitness.

COMMUNITY THERAPIES AND COUNSELING

The intellectual and emotional recovery of stroke survivors relies upon closely on supportive remedy and counselling. Counselling periods offer a steady and provoking putting for human beings to precise their feelings, communicate approximately troubles, and examine coping mechanisms. Additionally useful in enhancing intellectual well-being and reducing tension and despair are recuperation processes like pet treatment, track remedy, and artwork therapy. These interventions are seeking out to help stroke survivors' restoration techniques thru manner of addressing their specific intellectual requirements.

Chapter 14: Cognitive Rehabilitation

The desired rehabilitation method for humans who have had a stroke need to encompass cognitive rehabilitation. Memory, consciousness, trouble-fixing, and selection-making capabilities can all be adversely impacted by the use of cognitive problems brought on through using a stroke. This article examines masses of cognitive rehabilitation topics, together with comprehending cognitive troubles following a stroke, memory and interest training, desire-making and trouble-solving abilities, and techniques for enhancing elegant cognitive characteristic.

AFTER A STROKE, COGNITIVE DIFFICULTIES

Multiple cognitive issues may also furthermore result from a stroke, that can impair the brain's normal function. Memory,

attention, authorities feature, language, and visuospatial capabilities problems are commonplace cognitive impairments following a stroke. An person's capacity to carry out everyday duties, interact with others, and regain independence can all be extensively impacted through the ones issues. In order to create inexperienced rehabilitation plans and interventions, it's far essential to understand and apprehend those cognitive problems.

ASSISTANCE WITH MEMORY AND ATTENTION

The most not unusual cognitive troubles following a stroke encompass memory and hobby issues. Targeted education to decorate reminiscence and attention competencies is regularly blanketed in cognitive rehabilitation packages. Working reminiscence bodily sports, the usage of mnemonic gadgets, normal workout to extend attention spans, and techniques for sustaining interest and interest can also all be used to reap this. Additionally, compensatory techniques can help humans control reminiscence and interest troubles, together with the utilization of outside memory aids or the implementation of scheduled sporting events.

DECISION-MAKING AND PROBLEM-SOLVING SKILLS

Problem-fixing and preference-making skills may be impacted via cognitive deficits delivered on through a stroke. Through systematic problem-solving education, humans are assisted through using occupational therapists and cognitive rehabilitation experts in regaining those capabilities. This need to entail teaching preference-making frameworks, encouraging logical reasoning, encouraging purpose-directed questioning, and breaking down complicated sports activities into manageable elements. Individuals can restore independence and self assurance in their every day lives thru enhancing their problem-solving and selection-making skills.

METHODS TO IMPROVE COGNITIVE FUNCTION

After a stroke, there are various strategies that can be used to beautify popular cognitive feature. These encompass intellectual sports activities that stimulate cognitive talents, which includes puzzles, thoughts-education apps, and reminiscence video games. It has moreover been confirmed that bodily interest has high-quality impacts on cognitive not unusual performance. Furthermore, upholding a healthy way of life that consists of appropriate nutrients, sufficient sleep, strain manipulate, and social involvement promotes cognitive health and hurries up recuperation.

Chapter 15: Nutritional Support For Stroke Recovery

The healing and rehabilitation of these who have had a stroke depends closely on nutritional assist. In order to decorate commonplace health, speed up the recuperation method, and avoid complications, proper vitamins is vital. The important additives of dietary assist for stroke recuperation are examined in this text, which includes the know-how of the feature of nutrients, healthy ingesting guidelines, dietary problems unique to stroke survivors, and coping with swallowing troubles.

KNOWING THE PURPOSE OF NUTRITION

Through the supply of essential vitamins that aid mind feature, tissue restore, and widespread well being, nutrients performs a critical function within the restoration from a stroke. A balanced food regimen allows coronary heart fitness, blood stress control, ldl cholesterol manage, blood sugar manage, and retaining a wholesome weight. The recovery way for stroke survivors is aided through good enough weight loss plan, which moreover improves immunological characteristic and encourages large recuperation.

GUIDELINES FOR HEALTHY EATING

For stroke survivors to maximize their nutrient intake, they should adhere to healthful eating pointers. Generally speaking, the ones recommendations propose for ingesting pretty a few end result, veggies, complete grains, lean proteins, and healthy fat. For the control of cardiovascular fitness, limiting the consumption of saturated fat, trans fats, ldl ldl cholesterol, sodium, and brought sugars is important. For retaining large fitness and warding off problems, exact enough water is likewise essential.

CONSIDERATIONS FOR NUTRITION FOR STROKESURVIVORS

Healthcare businesses may additionally moreover need to address particular dietary desires of stroke survivors. These elements embody preserving an eye on and dealing with dietary constraints delivered on thru comorbid situations like diabetes, high blood strain, or dyslipidaemia. To encourage bowel regularity and prevent constipation, it's crucial to consume sufficient fibber. In order to manipulate dysphagia or swallowing problems and make certain they get the right nutrients with out jeopardizing their safety, stroke survivors might also moreover need to make nutritional adjustments.

HOW TO CONTROL SWALLOWING DIFFICULTIES

After a stroke, swallowing problems, additionally called dysphagia, can also arise and contact for precise care. Dietitians and speech-language pathologists are crucial in figuring out how properly people can swallow and making suggestions for modifications to the texture and consistency of food and drink. Changing to a mild or pureed diet, eating thickened liquids, or the use of unique swallowing techniques can be essential. In order to govern swallowing stressful situations and sell constant and amusing ingesting memories, it's miles essential to hold appropriate hydration and avoid aspiration.

Chapter 16: Assistive Technology And Home Modifications

In order to promote independence and decorate first-class of life for people with impairments or mobility problems, assistive technology and house versions are vital. These interventions looking for to deal with useful limits, boom accessibility, and assist people with sports of every day residing. The use of generation for unbiased living is included in this text together with great essential components of assistive generation and house adjustments, which incorporates mobility aids, accessibility domestic adjustments, and adaptive aids for every day residing.

ASSISTIVE TECHNOLOGIES FOR DAILY LIVING

Adaptive aids are gear or portions of system that help humans perform each day obligations extra independently. These aids may be modified own family device, dressing aids, bathing aids, reaches, seize bars, and adaptable kitchenware. In order to growth independence and protection in every day sports activities, occupational therapists are critical in evaluating someone's useful abilities and prescribing the satisfactory adaptive system.

TECHNOLOGIES THAT ASSIST MOBILITY

In order to help people with confined mobility circulate round and hold their balance, mobility resource devices have been created. These aids may additionally moreover embody wheelchairs, mobility scooters, walkers, crutches, and canes. A person's unique desires are assessed with the resource of occupational and bodily therapists, who then propose the first-rate mobility useful aid primarily based totally mostly on such things as electricity, stability, and sensible targets. To assure the high-quality use of those gadgets, proper turning into, schooling, and non-forestall help are crucial.

ACCESSIBILITY MODIFICATIONS TO HOMES

Making physical changes to the residing region is known as "home amendment," and it's far completed to increase accessibility and safety. For the ones who've mobility issues, this may entail which include ramps or stairlifts, enlarging entrances to residence wheelchairs, placing snatch bars and handrails in restrooms, and enhancing lights and evaluation for those who have sight impairments. To look at a person's desires and provide specialized adjustments that enhance accessibility and encourage impartial residing, occupational therapists, architects, and home trade professionals art work together.

TELECOMMUNICATIONS FOR INDEPENDENT LIVING

The potential of people with disabilities to live independently has considerably benefited by way of using technological enhancements. There are many remarkable assistive technology to be had, which include voice-activated smart home systems, environmental control gadgets, wearable fitness and protection video show gadgets, verbal exchange aids for humans with speech impairments, and specialised computer software program program and apps for reinforcing accessibility. In order to beautify someone's independence, productivity, and participation in each day sports activities, occupational therapists and assistive technology professionals collaborate to assess someone's wishes, deliver schooling and help, and suggest the tremendous technology.

Chapter 17: Managing Secondary Complications

Since people who have had a stroke may additionally increase pretty a few physical and sensory problems that would notably have an effect on their great of lifestyles, managing secondary complications is an critical part of stroke rehabilitation. In particular, this newsletter specializes in located up-stroke ache and sensory problems, exhaustion and sleep disturbances, bladder and bowel manipulate, and sexual characteristic as essential areas of managing secondary symptoms and signs after a stroke.

POST-STROKE DISCOMFORT AND SENSORY PROBLEMS

Some human beings ought to probable have ache after a stroke or sensory problems like numbness, tingling, or hypersensitive reaction. In order to create tailor-made interventions, healthcare specialists, which include neurologists and bodily therapists, compare the type and location of ache or sensory abnormalities. These can also moreover embody methods for handling drug remedies, ache control techniques, bodily treatment techniques to decorate sensation, and sensory re-schooling sports activities activities. People can growth their popular degree of consolation and engagement in every day sports by means of the usage of the usage of resolving those issues.

DISTURBANCES TO SLEEP AND FATIGUE

After a stroke, fatigue and sleep troubles are common subsequent consequences. Physical exertion, cognitive needs, and emotional pressure are a number of the issues occupational therapists and distinctive healthcare experts analyse and cope with even as treating patients for fatigue. They offer techniques for timing pastime, emphasizing relaxation periods, and maintaining electricity. Sleep hygiene practices, rest sporting activities, and treating underlying troubles like sleep apnea can all assist manage sleep disruptions. Enhancing common properly-being and enhancing rehabilitation results are achieved via manner of handling fatigue and getting higher sleep.

BOWEL AND BLADDER MANAGEMENT

Because of the neurological harm on account of a stroke, bladder and bowel issues can growth. For inexperienced bladder and bowel control, healthcare professionals such as urologists and rehabilitation experts study the affected person and offer answers. This may additionally furthermore entail developing a toileting time table, coping with medicinal pills, doing pelvic ground physical sports, and converting one's weight loss plan. To encourage independence and safety, assistive gadgets like higher bathroom seats or commodes may be counseled. Controlling bowel and bladder characteristic will growth consolation, lowers the threat of issues, and increases desired top notch of existence.

SEXUAL ACTIVITY FOLLOWING A STROKE

Sexual characteristic may be impacted with the aid of a stroke due to bodily, sensory, or emotional modifications. Professionals in the medical region, which consist of neurologists and counsellors, cope with troubles with sexual feature and offer assist and knowledge. The manage of medicinal capsules, counselling for emotional adjustment, studies of other varieties of intimacy, and adaptive sexual interest methods are just a few examples of interventions. To treat sexual function problems and decorate human beings's stylish well being, open verbal exchange, addressing mental reasons, and integrating partners inside the rehabilitation manner are vital.

Chapter 18: What Is Stroke And Causes?

A stroke, additionally known as a cerebrovascular twist of fate (CVA), is a scientific condition that takes area while blood go with the flow to part of the thoughts is disrupted or decreased. This interruption of blood supply can damage or ruin thoughts cells indoors minutes, important to the impairment of severa physical abilities managed thru the affected area of the brain.

Strokes may be labeled into foremost types:

The number one varieties of strokes are intracerebral hemorrhage (bleeding in the mind) and subarachnoid hemorrhage (bleeding inside the space most of the brain and the tissues defensive it).

Ischemic Stroke: This is the maximum not unusual form of stroke, accounting for approximately 85% of all instances. It takes vicinity whilst a blood clot or a plaque buildup interior a blood vessel blocks or narrows the artery offering blood to the brain.

The lack of blood flow deprives the thoughts cells of oxygen and vitamins, causing them to malfunction or die.

Hemorrhagic Stroke: This form of stroke takes place even as a blood vessel within the brain ruptures or leaks, number one to bleeding into or across the thoughts. Hemorrhagic strokes account for approximately 15% of all strokes but are typically extra severe and related to a higher hazard of disability or dying.

The symptoms and signs and symptoms of a stroke can range counting on the part of the mind affected but often encompass unexpected onset of:

Numbness or weak spot, commonly on one element of the body (face, arm, or leg)

Difficulty speaking or understanding speech.

Confusion or hassle with comprehension.

Vision troubles in a unmarried or every eyes.

Dizziness, loss of stability, or coordination problems.

Severe headache without a obvious motive.

It is vital to understand the signs and symptoms of a stroke and is trying to find right away clinical interest, as early intervention can considerably decorate the possibilities of healing.

Emergency treatment for a stroke may also involve remedy to dissolve blood clots (inside the case of an ischemic stroke) or surgical operation to prevent bleeding and restore broken blood vessels (in the case of a hemorrhagic stroke).

Rehabilitation and ongoing care are frequently essential to useful resource recuperation and control any lengthy-term results of a stroke.

Risk Factors of Stroke

Hypertension (excessive blood strain) is the most large risk element for stroke. It damages blood vessels and will increase the probability of blood clots or ruptures. Smoking, immoderate alcohol consumption and illicit drug use can make contributions to the threat of stroke.

Medical situations along with diabetes, excessive ldl ldl ldl cholesterol, atrial annoying infection (an strange heartbeat), and certain cardiovascular illnesses boom the risk of stroke.

Age is a hazard hassle, because the risk of stroke increases with advancing age.

Family records of stroke or genetic factors can predispose humans to stroke.

Certain way of life factors, at the side of negative weight-reduction plan, sedentary way of lifestyles, weight problems, and pressure, can growth the threat of stroke.

Moreso, the outcomes of a stroke can range extensively counting on the severity and region of the brain damage. Some not unusual outcomes include:

Physical impairments: Weakness or paralysis of limbs on one side of the frame, issue with balance and coordination, muscle stiffness, and issues with swallowing or talking.

Cognitive difficulties: Memory issues, problem concentrating, decreased hassle-fixing capabilities, and challenges with comprehension and verbal exchange.

Emotional and mental modifications: Depression, anxiety, temper swings, and emotional instability can arise after a stroke.

Sensory adjustments: Loss or alteration of sensation in positive frame factors, together with numbness, tingling, or heightened sensitivity.

Changes in imaginative and prescient: Blurred or double visio Lost of imaginative and prescient in a single or every eyes, or field of regard defects.

Fatigue and sleep disturbances: Many stroke survivors enjoy fatigue that can drastically impact every day activities. Sleep problems, which encompass insomnia or sleep apnea, also can upward push up.

Recovery and Rehabilitation: Stroke rehabilitation is a critical part of the recovery tool. It hobbies to enhance functional talents and help people regain independence. Rehabilitation may additionally consist of:

Occupational remedy to regain talents essential for every day residing sports activities, together with dressing, consuming, and bathing.

Speech remedy to cope with speech and swallowing issues.

Cognitive remedy to assist with reminiscence, hobby, and trouble-fixing skills.

Psychological help to address emotional and mental disturbing situations.

Assistive gadgets or adaptive techniques to capture up on disabilities.

Chapter 19: How To Manage Stroke Patient

Help A Stroke Patient To Take Their Medications As Prescribe By Doctor: It is essential for the individual to take their drugs as prescribed with the useful resource in their healthcare corporation. This may additionally additionally furthermore encompass drugs to control their blood stress and save you blood clots. It is essential for the character to take their medicinal tablets as prescribed with the beneficial aid of their healthcare provider. This can also contain placing reminders, organizing their medicinal drug, and coordinating with their healthcare team to make certain that their drugs are strolling effectively.

Health Diet, Healthy Lifestyle, Regular Exersice Is a Basic Key for Quick Stroke Recovery: Helping the person to consume a healthful weight loss program and get normal exercise can help them get over their stroke and prevent destiny strokes.

It is likewise critical to be affected man or woman and knowledge, as recuperation from a stroke can be an extended and tough approach. If you feel beaten, do no longer hesitate to be trying to find useful resource from buddies, family, or a healthcare expert. A wholesome diet is crucial for stroke restoration and can assist the individual to regain their energy and strength. Encourage the man or woman to devour some of stop result, vegetables, entire grains, and lean proteins, and to restrict their consumption of salt, sugar, and threatening fat.

Help the character to control any ongoing scientific problems: Some human beings who have had a stroke may also moreover have ongoing clinical problems in conjunction with excessive blood strain, diabetes, or coronary coronary heart illness. Help the person to manipulate the ones situations through encouraging them to examine their remedy plan and searching for scientific hobby as wanted.

Stroke Patient Needs Encouragement: Encourage the character to be as impartial as possible and to take part in their own recuperation. This can help them feel extra on pinnacle of factors and decorate their conceitedness.

Safe And Spacious Environment Is Essential: Remove any tripping risks or different capacity safety risks from the person's living region. Make positive they have got cushty and without difficulty reachable seating, and take into account putting in handrails inside the rest room to help them get round.

Every Caregiver Also Need Support For Prevent A Burnout: If you are the number one caregiver for a person who has had a stroke, it may be bodily and emotionally annoying. Don't be afraid to invite for assist from friends, own family, or expert caregivers. This can assist save you caregiver burnout and ensure that the individual receiving care is getting the manual they need. Caring for someone who has had a stroke can be a difficult enjoy. Don't be afraid to are seeking out assist from pals, circle of relatives, or a healthcare expert in case you are feeling beaten. It is critical to attend to your very own bodily and emotional well-being as properly.

Be Familiar with Person's Condition and Treatments: Keep song of the person's development and any changes of their situation. This will help you recognize what to anticipate and a manner to exceptional assist their recovery.

Every Stroke Caregivers Need Support Recourses: Caring for someone who has had a stroke may be a hard experience. There are many resources to be had to help caregivers deal with the wishes of care giving and locate assist. Don't hesitate to obtain out to organizations which include the Stroke Association or the National Caregivers Association for help and useful useful resource.

Every Stroke Patient Needs Easy Movement-Transportation: If the person is not capable of pressure because of their stroke, you could need to assist them with transportation to appointments and unique sports activities. This may additionally moreover involve riding them yourself or coordinating with public transportation or trip-sharing services.

Assist with economic subjects: Depending on the severity of the stroke, the man or woman might also want assist dealing with their fee variety. This may additionally contain paying bills, managing financial institution bills, and organizing their monetary files.

www.ingramcontent.com/pod-product-compliance
Lightning Source LLC
Chambersburg PA
CBHW051728020426
42333CB00014B/1211